SEX AND YOUR DIET

May all your
mastications be
prophylactic!
Candy Cummings

SEX AND YOUR DIET

BY CANDY CUMMING, M.S., R.D.

LEISURE PRESS

Champaign, Illinois

Published by Leisure Press
A division of Human Kinetics Publishers, Inc.
Box 5076
Champaign, IL 61820

ISBN: 0-88011-166-6

Cover and book design: Brian Groppe
Cartoons: David Hebenstreit
Illustrations: John Jett
Typesetting: Lewis Publishing, Oakland, California

Library of Congress Cataloging in Publication Date

Cumming, Candy.
Sex and your diet.

Bibliography: p.
Includes index.
1. Generative organs—Diseases—Nutritional aspects.
2. Sex (Biology)—Nutritional aspects. 3. Vitamin A—
Physiological effect. 4. Vitamin therapy. 5. Minerals
in human nutrition. I. Title.
RC881.C953 1986 616.6'5 83-80738
ISBN 0-88011-166-6

Dedication

To "T" and "P" and a good
buddy whose friendships
have meant a lot to me.

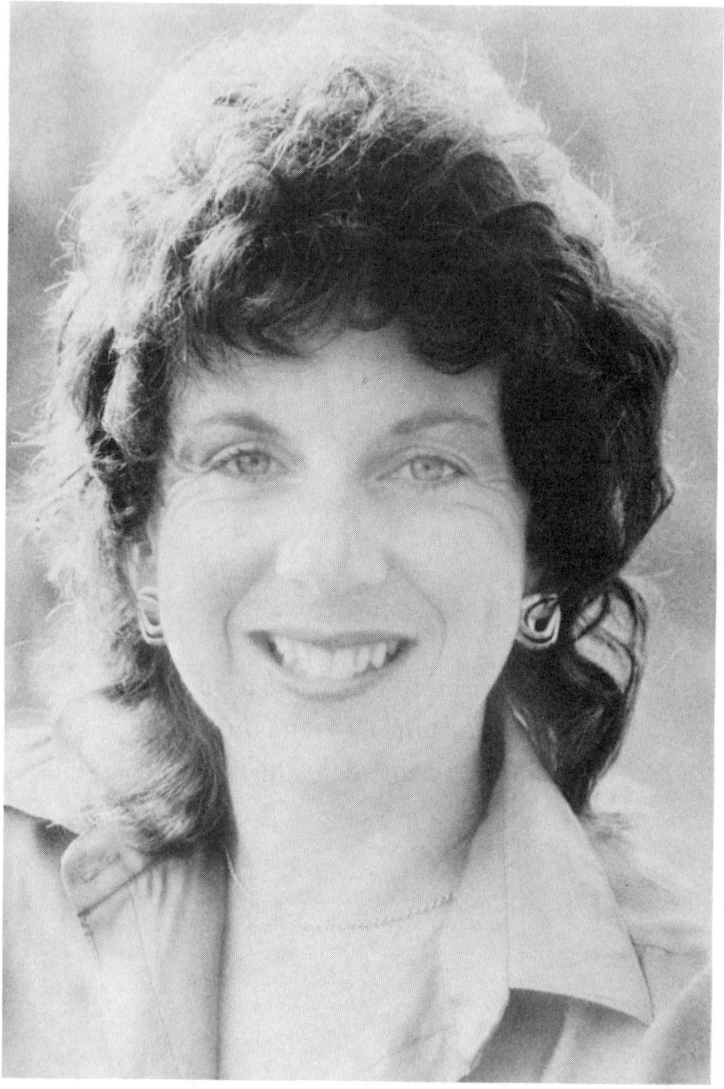

Candy Cumming, M.S., R.D. is a nutrition consultant to several of America's major corporations. Specializing in health promotion, she is a prolific public speaker and regularly appears on television and radio talk shows, including The Merv Griffin Show. She earned her graduate degree in Nutrition and Public Health from Columbia University. Subsequently, she worked as a dietician for the Albert Einstein College of Medicine in Bronx, N.Y. and then as a clinical nutritionist for the University of California at San Diego Medical Center. She is the author of the best selling book, *An Eator's Guide: Nutrition Basics for Busy People,* and has written numerous articles on nutrition for a variety of national magazines. In 1977 the American Dietetic Association recognized her as the "Young Dietician of the Year." Currently, she resides in San Diego, California.

CONTENTS

ACKNOWLEDGMENTS

The help and support of many friends helped create *"Carrot."* An especially big thank-you goes to Cindy Knott, who did a lot of footwork for me. A whole bunch of carrot-supporters deserve the same. Thanks, everyone: Phil Anderson; "Bommy"; Herb Boynton; Kate Burns; Ellen Coleman; Rick, LaVera, Sean and Kirk Cumming; Carol Fisk; Mary Furey; Paul Gerard; Marty Granger; Barbara Haggarty; Barbara Kass; Joyce Knott; Miriam Lamb; Sue and Jim Peterson; Mark McCarty; Vicky Newman; Steve and Martha Richardson; Jane and Neal Wadler; Jeff Layng; Jim White; and the makers of my Apple Computer!

INTRODUCTION

With a name like Candy Cumming, I figure that a book about food and sex is in my destiny. I have always been interested in food. As for sex, interest in that came a wee bit later. In my many nutrition classes food was always discussed, and the sex-talk was saved and savored elsewhere. But surely there's a connection between food and sex.

The ancients thought so. They considered many foods aphrodisiacs, heighteners of the sexual experience. Yet for most of us the quality of our sexual experiences may be diminished because of a lack of good health, not because of a lack of aphrodisiacs. Being sick, tired and headachey has probably done more to quell sexual desire/ability than any aphrodisiac has ever stimulated it.

Obviously any illness can interfere with our sex lives. Yet in scanning the recent medical literature it appears that nutritional factors profoundly influence our sexual health, too! What we eat does affect our sexuality. That's why I decided to write this book.

A Nutritional Guide to Human Sexuality is a brief, simplified review of some recent findings in the food-sex connection. It is the first time a lot of this information has come together in one volume. It is not a treatment manual and should not be used in that way. It's meant to remind us that we need to eat wholesome, basic foods daily. You'll soon appreciate that there's no place for nutrient-depleted foods.

A lot of tables listing the nutritional contents of food are included, because good nutritional habits are built, first and foremost, on good eating habits. At certain times and under certain conditions (and preferably under the guidance of a knowledgeable physician or registered dietitian), nutritional supplements may be helpful in augmenting nutritional intake—but they are no replacement for good, wholesome, delicious food. Eating, like sex, is a sensual experience. Food is meant to be savored and enjoyed. Anyone who thinks nutrition is only available in tablet form should probably also invent an orgasma-pill. Just as the caress of a loving partner nurtures you, healthful foods "love" you from within by supplying you with life's most basic essentials.

By no means will proper nutrition straighten out all your sexual difficulties. However, healthful foods do provide many factors that preserve your health, including various aspects of your sexuality. Good eating habits can avert your feeling sick, tired and headachey, too. The role of diet, once overlooked and now being explored, is certainly worthy of some consideration.

Sexuality is an extremely complex issue. Nutrition has its place among many factors that influence it. Whether or not aphrodisiacs heighten sexual experience doesn't really matter—chances are that healthy lovers who can communicate with and enjoy one another are their own best aphrodisiacs after all!

Some chapters target men's issues; others feature factors of concern to women. If you are sincerely interested in getting all the benefits good food has to offer your sex life, read the whole book—after all, it takes two to tango. Besides, then you can get into mutual mastication.

I'll leave you with the book now. It's time for me to eat my carrot!

1

SEX AND THE SINGLE CARROT

You may be wondering about the connection between carrots and your love life. Come on now, put your kinky thoughts away. If you want to maintain your sexual vitality, this is not a subject to be in the dark about. And, speaking of the dark . . .

Carrots, as the old saying goes, help you see in the dark. This certainly enhances your sex life if you prefer nighttime love making. Assuming that a glimpse of your partner during love play heightens your pleasure, carrots could be considered a kind of secondary aphrodisiac. Still, carrots do more than assure "love at first sight" in the night.

High in vitamin A, carrots are a great protector of your epithelial tissues. In case you are unfamiliar with this kind of tissue, it is not a fancy form of Kleenex. Rather, it's in the stuff on the outside of your body: your skin. Epithelial tissue also forms the linings of internal body parts that have a connection to the outside world—this includes your lungs, mouth, esophagus, stomach, intestines, vagina and cervix (if you have them) and the prostate (if you have that instead). It stands to reason that if any of these parts are not well, your sexual activity may diminish. But have you ever considered that what you eat can help shape the health of your "private parts"? And wouldn't you agree that healthy parts are vital for physically expressing your love?

That some everyday foods contribute to the well-being of your sex life should be happy news. And I hope it is for you! But it's not for many people. You see, the sad thing about vitamin A-rich foods is that a lot of people eat too little of them. During the last two major nutritional surveys in our country, it was discovered that a substantial number of people consumed less than recommended amounts. That doesn't mean that people are starving to death. It does mean, however, that they are making some poor food choices and, probably, forgetting to munch on fruits and vegetables each day. If you beat it out the door in the morning and grab a doughnut along the way, hit up a fast-food joint or brown bag a sandwich at lunch, you'll be low in vitamin A unless you manage to toss in a salad, a few vegetables and/or a piece of fruit sometime during the day. The Recommended Dietary Allowance for vitamin A is 5,000 IU daily. That may sound like a tall order, but to see how little it takes to get so much, see Table 1-1.

Rather than glancing at the chart, take out a pen or pencil and circle the foods on the list that you ate yesterday. To figure out how much vitamin A you got, you'll also need to consider how much of each food you ate. It says one carrot has 5,000 IU; if you ate two, then double the figure. If you ate a skimpy carrot stick, you may have only gotten a fifth of a portion, etc. If yesterday was a bum day for "A," then it's possible you picked up a lot on another day. What I suggest is to keep track of your intake for a week. If your score totals at least 35,000 IU in seven days, you're doing great. If you didn't get up that high, then mark an "X" alongside foods you like (or are willing to try) and stock up on them. I have found that although people like some foods, they often forget to eat them. There are quite a few people who eat only one serving of vegetables a day. This is often iceberg lettuce, crunchy and conveniently served in most restaurants, but with a pretty low vitamin A content.

As you can see from the chart, all it takes is one carrot a day, a tiny investment that can pay off big dividends. Carrots are relatively inexpensive or easily grown in a backyard, so there's no reason for anyone to be without one. When you stop to think about it, a good carrot is a lot easier to find than a good lover! But it's best to have both, one for good loving and the other to keep your loving parts in good condition.

If you're low on A, some of your "sexy" parts can eventually become "horny." In medical mumbo jumbo, "horny" means that your epithelial tissues have undergone changes, that mucous-secreting cells have become dry or "scaly," or "keratinized." Unfortunately these changes are pre-cancerous and can be brought about by an inadequate intake of vitamin A. If your doctor were writing this in medical jargon, you would see something that looked like "squamous metaplasia" (provided you could read his handwriting!). When this abnormal tissue replaces the healthy stuff, there are grounds for suspecting an increased risk of cancer. Sounds alarming, doesn't it? Well, it is! But what's astounding is the fact that this metaplasia can be inhibited by an adequate intake of vitamin A!

Table 1-1: Vitamin A Content of Foods Rich in Beta-carotene*
Recommended Dietary Allowance:
5,000 IU
6,000 IU if pregnant
8,000 IU if breastfeeding

FOOD	SERVING	IU/SERVING
Fruits:		
Apricots	2-3 medium	2700
Canteloupe	1/4	3400
Mango	½	4800
Melon balls	1 cup	3540
Nectarines	2	1650
Papaya	1/3	1750
Peaches	1 cup	2240
Plums, purple	2	1250
Prunes	4	760
Pumpkin, canned	2/5 cup	6400
Watermelon	1/16 of a 10″ × 16″ melon	5310
Vegetables:		
Asparagus	1 cup	1485
Beet greens, cooked	½ cup	6100
Broccoli	1 stalk, 5″ long	3500
Carrot, raw	1 small	5000
Carrots, cooked	2/3 cup	15000
Chard, raw	3/5 cup	6500
Collards	½ cup	6500
Dandelion greens, cooked	½ cup	14000
Kale, cooked	¾ cup	8900
Romaine	3½ oz	1900
Peas & carrots	1 cup	14880
Spinach, cooked	½ cup	7500
Squash, winter, cooked	½ cup	4200
Squash, acorn	½	2640
Squash, butternut, cooked	1 cup mashed	13230
Sweet potato	5 oz	14900
Tomato	1 large, raw	1800
Tomato sauce, canned	½ cup	1650
Turnip greens, cooked	½ cup	7600

*Beta-carotene is a form of vitamin A that appears to be helpful in reducing cancer risk when eaten in adequate amounts.

Adapted from:
Pennington, J. A., Church, H. N. *Bowes and Church's Food Values of Portions Commonly Used*, Philadphia: J. B. Lippincott Company, 1980.

Studies of mice and men bear this out. Research on laboratory animals has repeatedly shown that too little vitamin A increases cancer susceptibility. In humans it has been observed that when blood vitamin A levels are low, cancer incidence is high. As you know, smokers have a very high risk of lung cancer compared with non-smokers, but the smokers at highest risk are those with low blood levels of vitamin A. Your blood levels of vitamin A can sink below a healthy level if you avoid vitamin A-rich foods (especially green and yellow fruits and vegetables) over an extended period of time. You'd better take another look at 1-1.

When it comes to cancer of the prostate, many studies have been done on both mice and men. Several nutritional factors appear to influence the course of prostate cancer (especially dietary fat, which will be covered in another chapter). But one epidemiological survey in Japan strongly suggests that green and yellow vegetables make for healthier prostates. In this study of over 100,000 men, it was found that a high intake of colorful vegetables was correlated with a low mortality rate from prostate cancer. The epidemiologist who reviewed the data suggested that this vegetable intake may help explain why Japan has just about the lowest incidence of prostate cancer mortality while the U.S. has nearly the highest. Japanese men who were protected from prostate cancer ate twice as many green and yellow vegetables when compared to the typical American, yet the incidence of prostate cancer mortality is five to six times higher among American whites than among Japanese. American blacks, on the other hand, have double the risk of whites! At this point, carrots probably never looked so good!

Even mouse prostates depend on vitamin A. Laboratory scientists have performed experiments that demonstrate a protective role for vitamin A in prostate tissue. Here's what they did: They got some mice. Then they had to find their itty bitty prostates, which they removed and placed in a culture medium. Next they applied a chemical carcinogen, and sure enough, precancerous changes began to take place. However, when they simultaneously administered vitamin A, the precancerous changes were inhibited and reversed! This study along with the epidemiological study in Japan strongly suggests that an adequate intake of vitamin A can be helpful in reducing your risk of prostate cancer.

Vitamin A also plays a protective role in women. Female hamsters whose chow has been supplemented with vitamin A do not get cervical cancer, even if scientists introduce a chemical carcinogen to the cervix. Do you have anything in common with hamsters? Probably. A recent report correlated a low consumption of vitamin A and beta-carotene (the precursor of vitamin A in fruits and vegetables) among women who had cervical dysplasia. (Dysplasia means that the tissue is developing abnormally.) In addition, the researchers also found that a specific vitamin A-containing protein was either absent or minimally detectable in the cervical tissue that had undergone the most dysplasia.

Whether you're male or female, a carrot a day helps ensure the normal growth of the tissues that make up your sexual parts. As such, it can protect you from developing cancer.

To understand how a carrot or most dietary factors influence the course of cancer development, you need to know a little bit about the cancer process. Briefly, cancer develops in two-stages. The first stage is called the initiation phase, during which time mutagenic (abnormal) changes take place within the cell. At this point you may have a few cancerous cells. What happens during the next phase will determine whether or not you develop the diagnosable disease. This second phase, called the promotional phase, can last 30 years or more. Vitamin A apparently blocks the progression of cancer during the promotional phase. That's why it is protective. On the other hand, an excessive consumption of dietary fat hastens the development of certain cancers (prostate, breast, uterus, colon and rectum.) Substances that spur cancer growth during this second stage of cancer development are called "promoters."

While the Japanese have a lower mortality rate from prostate cancer, they have the same incidence of "latent" cancer as that of people in high mortality areas. Apparently something in the environment blocks the development of this small number of cancer cells into full-blown disease. The Japanese diet is high in one protective factor, vitamin A, and low in fat, a promotional factor. The American diet, unfortunately, is exactly the opposite. High in fat and low in vitamin A, our national diet only tends to encourage cancer growth.

All this exciting news about vitamin A may make you come to a few faulty conclusions. One is that vitamin A cures cancer. It can prevent or halt its development, but it doesn't cure it per se so it's not a good idea to play doctor with yourself, or anyone else for that matter. Good nutrition is an essential component of therapy, but not a replacement for it. The point is this: If you eat an adequate amount of green and yellow vegetables, you will lessen your susceptibility to cancer.

Another erroneous conclusion you might make is to load yourself up with vitamin A supplements. Yet it is a fat-soluble vitamin and is stored in the body; daily dosing with excessive amounts can eventually produce dangerously high levels. This problem is most common in people getting 20-30 times the RDA, for dermatological conditions. When "hypervitaminosis A" occurs, you become nauseated, vomit a lot, have blurred vision and intense headaches. Damage to your liver, bone and blood cells also takes place. Besides, there is the possibility that too much vitamin A could hurt your sex life! Rat studies indicate that large doses can cause testicle abnormalities that lead to a decrease in testicle mass, but whether or not this is true for humans is still unknown.

Excessive dosing with vitamin A can spell trouble for pregnant women. Not long ago a woman who had been taking a daily dose of 150,000 IU of vitamin A during the early part of her pregnancy gave birth to a child with multiple malformations of the central nervous system. The baby died shortly after being born. The problem was considered to be related to the high dosage of vitamin A.

You may not be a "pill freak" and pop vitamins, but you may want to eat everything orange in sight. I once had a patient who was drinking carrot juice by the carloads. She loved peaches, yams, canteloupes and apricots. She ate so much yellow food that she turned yellow! At first glance she looked as if she had jaundice, but her diet history showed that she went overboard on foods high in carotene (the precursor of vitamin A, and what also imparts the orange color). By cutting down drastically on these foods, she eventually regained her normal color. A recent report also highlights the wisdom in that old pearl about "too much of a good thing." Women eating large quantities of carotene-rich vegetables developed carotenemia, an abnormal elevation in blood carotene levels. Along with this came menstrual irregularities. After reducing the amount of dietary carotene, their blood levels returned to normal and their menstrual periods resumed. One woman followed the advice for a while and experienced good results—unil she reverted to her former eating style. Sure enough, her blood carotene levels zoomed up and she failed to menstruate!

Obviously the point is not to overdo it. The other point is not to underdo it either. Vitamin A is readily available from ordinary foods that you can easily eat each day. Making sure your dietary intake is adequate is a simple way to lessen your risk of certain forms of cancer. If you also happen to use a vitamin A supplement, it's a good idea to keep your total intake (from food and supplementary sources combined) somewhere between 5000 and 25,000 IU a day.

In looking back over Table 1-1, you can see that it doesn't take a Herculean effort to eat what you need. All it takes is one carrot a day. Since that carrot provides enough vitamin A to protect your vital sexy parts, you might say that sex is better with a single carrot!

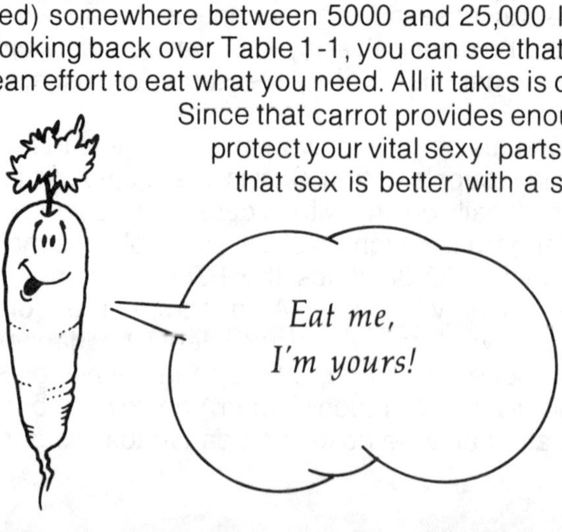

2

SEXY MOUTH

Man meets woman. In the movies it's usually over a drink and, more often than not, a cigarette. They become enchanted with each other's charms. Several drinks and cigarettes later, they may be kissing and . . . ! What the unsuspecting couple doesn't realize is that the drinks and weeds that accompanied their getting into action may eventually take them out of action. Booze and butts (as in cigarettes) are not sexy!

If you're into kissing and/or any kind of oral gratification, then it's a good idea to ease up on the spirits (or quit drinking if you're a heavy drinker) and kick your smoking habits as well. The problem is that people who are heavily into smoking and alcohol are setting the stage for cancer, specifically cancer of the oral cavity, including the mouth, esophagus and naso-larynx. Somehow I get the picture that a sick mouth doesn't lend itself to amorous interludes. Even though your love may be stronger than ever, there is no sense in jeopardizing your ability to demonstrate it with a kiss.

Epidemiologists, who study factors contributing to diseases, repeatedly find an association between chronic alcohol consumption (meaning a lot of booze, frequently, as opposed to a few social drinks occasionally), smoking and these head and neck cancers. Because heavy drinkers are often heavy smokers scientists are having a tough time assessing the contribution of each factor independently. But when they're together, the evidence is clear. Surveys in the United States also highlight this fact. In Utah, where per capita use of alcohol and tobacco is well below the national average, the incidence of cancer of the esophagus is much lower than that of the rest of the country. Men, who traditionally smoke more and drink more than women, succomb more often to head and neck cancers than women do. This further supports the existing evidence that the combination of booze and butts heightens cancer risk.

While smoking and drinking are major factors involved, they are not the only ones. Certain nutritional deficiencies also seem to contribute. So do contaminants of certain grains, and opium. This may help explain why esophageal cancer is endemic in certain areas of the world. There is a region in China called the "esophageal cancer belt" where the incidence of this disease runs high, particularly among people born in the Fukkien Province. To date, clinical investigations indicate that the nutritional factors presumed to play a major role include deficiencies of both vitamin A and riboflavin (vitamin B-2). Interestingly, alcohol interferes with both of these nutrients.

Nobody really knows exactly how alcohol, cigarettes, cigars, or pipe and chewing tobacco lead to cancer. But it looks as if tobacco and/or tobacco smoke supply carcinogenic material that initiate the process. And alcohol appears to act as a promoter—speeding up the appearance of the disease. Not only do heavy drinkers usually have miserable diets, their spirited beverage also impairs the absorption and/or heightens urinary excretion of many nutrients. This makes an already poor diet a whole lot worse. A recent Department of Health and Human Services publication noted that cancers of the head and neck seem to occur most commonly in people who do not eat nutritionally balanced diets—so a drinking habit superimposed upon lousy eating habits is a double whammy!

Surveys show that American urban blacks have a higher risk than others in the States. Whether this reflects too much drinking or smoking and too little nutrition has not been spelled out. But it's interesting that blacks tend to have an intolerance to lactose, the sugar found in milk. With milk being a major provider of riboflavin, a diet without milk may easily lead to riboflavin deficiency. Inadequate dietary intakes of this nutrient have frequently been found among the urban poor. In several studies, a correlation was found between milk consumption and riboflavin status. (More milk meant better riboflavin status.) So if you're not a milk drinker, make sure you get some riboflavin. Liver, cheese, leafy vegetables, whole grain and enriched bread and cereals, legumes and sprouted seeds are also good sources. And be sure to keep these foods stored in dark places. Light destroys riboflavin. If you do buy milk, buy it in cartons and not in transparent plastic jugs.

One of the many functions of riboflavin is the maintenance of the epithelial tissues, and the skin and upper alimentary tract tissues appear to be especially vulnerable when there are low levels. In mice, a riboflavin-deficient diet leads to a progressive deterioration of the epithelium in the mouth and esophagus. Researchers who administer cancer-initiating substances to laboratory animals report that riboflavin deficiency speeds up the development of tumors. These studies, along with evidence of this disease among B-2-deficient human beings, show it's not a wise idea to "kiss off" foods rich in riboflavin—not if you want to keep your kisser kissing.

How does vitamin A enter the picture? Considering A's role in epithelial health, it's easy enough to understand why too little of it contributes to precancerous changes in the mouth and esophagus. But get this! Alcohol is capable of lowering vitamin A levels in the blood and could make an otherwise adequate diet deficient.

Alcohol has an additional effect that's more direct than its role in nutrient loss. As a solvent, alcohol may facilitate the passage of carcinogenic substances through membranes and into the cells of target tissues. Or it could be that exposure to alcohol causes an alteration within cells that activates the carcinogens in tobacco. The precise role(s) alcohol plays in head and neck cancers is still unknown. However, it is a cancer promoter and will hasten the onset of malignant disease.

Fortunately for your own protection, you do not have to wait for scientists to determine how alcohol hastens carcinogenesis. Just knowing that alcohol (especially when combined with a tobacco habit) contributes to cancer should provide you with enough incentive to lay off heavy boozing and butts. If you find yourself saying, "Yes, I'd like to do that, but . . ." remember that "but, but, but" sounds more like a stalling engine than someone interested in preserving a sexy mouth.

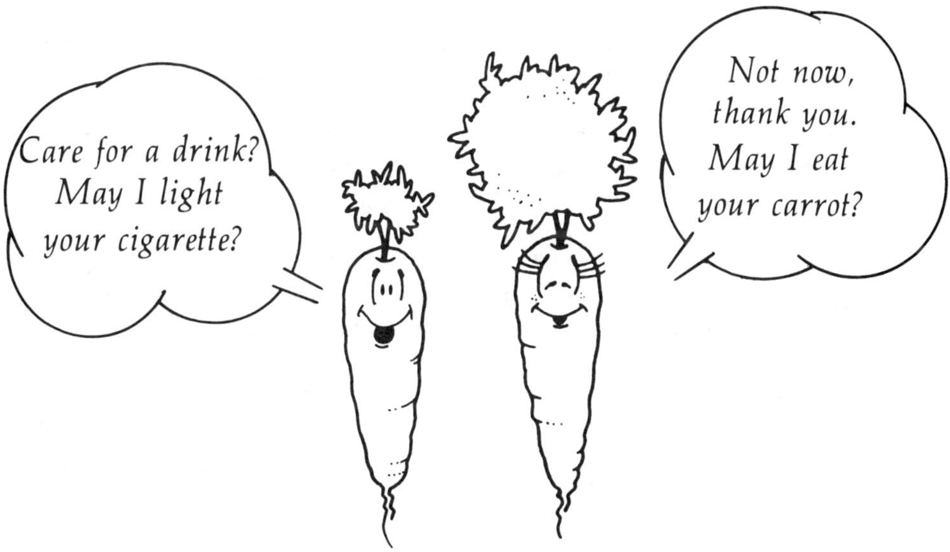
Care for a drink? May I light your cigarette?
Not now, thank you. May I eat your carrot?

3

HIGH-CLASS PAP

If you're a woman old enough to be reading this book, you have (I hope) had a number of Pap smears during your life. If you are embarrassed by pelvic exams, you are being too short-sighted. You see, a Pap smear can detect early signs of cervical cancer, the third most common cancer in women. (Breast and skin cancers rank as numbers one and two.)

The cervix, as you may or may not know, is the narrow lower and outer end of your uterus. It is located at the far end of your vaginal canal. Even by standing on your head and using a mirror, it's doubtful you could ever see your own. This area is very vulnerable to malignant changes, and that's why a yearly Pap smear is recommended. When taking a Pap smear, the physician gets a few cervical cells by using a cotton swab in the inner cervical canal leading to the uterus, and by scraping the outer portion of the cervix with a wooden spatula. It doesn't hurt, yet this simple test can detect 95% of early cervical abnormalities. This test alone has helped reduce the death rate from cervical cancer by more than 50%. Unfortunately a majority of women do not have a yearly Pap test! It has been estimated that if all women had this test annually, cervical cancer would be eliminated as a cause of death. If it's been over a year since you've been tested, why not call your physician and set up a visit right now? Even if this is my idea, don't resist it. After all, it's your cervix!

More than likely, you have heard about different classes of Pap smears. Basically here's how it is: The higher the class, the worse the problem. There's a big difference between a first-class Pap and a high-class one. Class I means there are no abnormal cells. In Class II, a few atypical cells are seen but these are believed to be caused by an inflammation. By the time a smear is Class III, cancer cells are suspected. But in both Classes IV and V cancer cells are definitely there. If your smear is Class III, IV or V, chances are your physician will do a few additional tests and/or a biopsy to find out what is really happening. Further treatment depends on what's discovered.

So far it looks as if cervical cancer is more common among

Figure 3-1: The Female Reproductive System

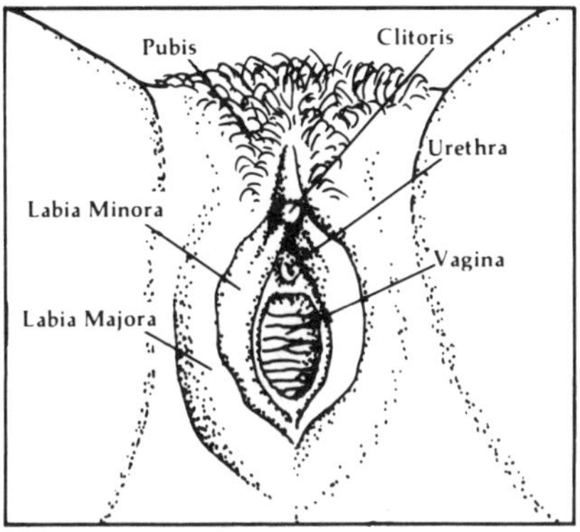

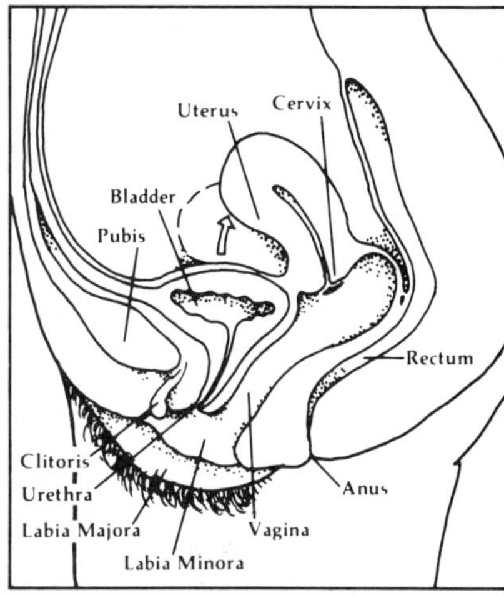

women from lower socioeconomic groups. In addition, women who began intercourse early are at higher risk than those who are "late bloomers." So are women who do "it" frequently as well as those who have multiple sexual partners. And, as mentioned in Chapter I, women whose diets are low in vitamin A are highly susceptible. This is not surprising, since most cervical cancer is the "squamous" kind.

However, it appears that another nutritional factor is also quite protective: vitamin C. This was accidently discovered during a recent study while scientists were seeking an explanation for the action of vitamin A. Women frequenting a clinic in a New York hospital participated in the study that included Pap smears, other tests, a diet history and nutritional analysis. Their findings were compatible with others that have shown a higher risk among the poor. In this study black women had more cervical abnormalities than white women. Even considering variables in sexual habits, they still found that vitamin C had its own unique effect on cervical health. Incidentally, their results also suggested that cervical dysplasia (abnormality) was more common among women whose diets were lower in beta/carotene, the precursor of vitamin A.

Black or white, women with cervical dysplasias were consuming half the amount of vitamin C as women who tested normal. Many of the women in the troubled group had intakes of vitamin C as low as 30 mg, half the daily recommended amount. When intake dipped to 30 mg or below, risk of cervical dysplasia skyrocketed! Interestingly, a low intake of vitamin C was associated with low income. Is this why poor women are at higher risk? Since vitamin C is abundant in fruits and vegetables, it's quite possible that these are omitted for one reason or another, perhaps because they are relatively expensive.

Poor or not, if you tend to skip fresh foods most of the time, you'd better reconsider your eating habits. Single people often have the

3-1: Vitamin C Content of Foods
Recommended Dietary Allowance:
60 mg
80 mg if pregnant
100 mg if breastfeeding

FOOD	SERVING SIZE	mg VITAMIN C
Asparagus, cooked	1 cup	40
Beans, green or yellow	1 cup	20
Beans, green or yellow, cooked	1 cup	15
Beet greens, cooked	½ cup	30
Broccoli, raw	1 stalk (3 oz)	110
Broccoli, cooked	2/3 cup	90
Broccoli, frozen, cooked	3½ oz	55
Brussels sprouts, cooked	6-7	85
Cabbage, Chinese, cooked	½ cup	25
Cabbage, common, raw	1 cup	50
Cabbage, cooked	1 cup	40
Cabbage, red, raw	1 cup	60
Cauliflower, raw	1 cup	80
Cauliflower, cooked	1 cup	60
Celery, raw	3 outer stalks	15
Chard, cooked	1 cup	50
Collards, cooked	½ cup	90
Dandelion greens, cooked	½ cup	35
Kale, cooked	1 cup	155
Kohlrabi, cooked	2/3 cup	45
Lettuce, romaine	3½ oz	20
Mustard greens, cooked	½ cup	50
Okra, cooked	8-9 pods	20
Parsley, raw, chopped	2 tablespoons	35
Peas, green, cooked	2/3 cup	20
Peppers, hot chili, mature red, raw	3½ oz	370
Peppers, green, raw	1 large	130
Potato, baked	1 (3½ oz)	20
Radish, red, raw	10	25
Rutabaga, raw	3½ oz	45
Rutabaga, cooked	½ cup	25
Spinach, raw	3½ oz	50
Spinach, cooked	½ cup	25
Squash, acorn, cooked; also butternut, hubbard	½	20
Sweet potato, baked	1 small	20
Tomato, red, ripe, raw	1 small	25
Tomato juice	1 large (6 oz)	45
Turnip greens, cooked	⅓ cup	140
Turnips, raw	¾ cup	35
Turnips, cooked	2/3 cup	20

Table 3-1 Continued, Vitamin C Content of Foods

FOOD	SERVING SIZE	mg VITAMIN C
Fruits and Juices:		
Apricots, raw	2-3	10
Banana, raw	1 large	20
Blackberries, raw	⅝ cup	20
Blueberries, raw	⅝ cup	15
Canteloupe, raw	¼ melon	35
Cherries, sweet, raw	15 large	10
Currants, black, raw	3½ oz	200
Grapefruit, raw	½	40
Grapefruit juice, fresh	½ cup	50
Grapefruit juice, canned	½ cup	35
Guava, common, raw	1 medium	240
Honeydew, raw	1 wedge, 2" wide	35
Lemon, raw, peeled	1	50
Lemon juice, fresh	¼ cup	30
Melon balls	1 cup	35
Nectarines	2 medium	15
Orange, raw, peeled	1 small	50
	1 large	120
Orange juice, fresh	1 cup	125
Orange juice, from frozen	1 cup	110
Orange juice, canned	1 cup	100
Papaya	1/3	50
Papaya juice,canned	½ cup	50
Peaches, raw	1 cup	10
Pineapple, raw	¾ cup	20
Raspberries, raw or frozen	¾ cup	25
Strawberries, raw	1 cup	90
Strawberries, frozen	½ cup	65
Tangelo	1 medium	25
Tangerine	1 large or 2 small	30
Watermelon	1 cup	15
Watermelon	1 slice (6" diam., 1½" thick)	40

Adapted from: Pennington, J.A., Church, H. N. *Bowes and Church's Food Values of Portions Commonly Used.* Philadelphia: J. B. Lippincott Company, 1980.

habit of not stocking up on fresh produce. I remember when I was single how many times I went out to dinner with friends, leaving bags of veggies in the refrigerator and finding bags of unidentifiable green glop a week later. If this is also your problem, then vegetables might not be the things to stockpile. Citrus fruits, melons and frozen OJ concentrate keep a lot better. You can also get fresh fruits (especially grapefruits and melon) at most eateries, and orange juice just about anywhere, including a bar!

Why vitamin C protects against the development of cervical cancer has yet to be spelled out. However, it plays a similar "guardian" role in other areas as well, including the stomach, colon and rectum. This is not all that surprising, because vitamin C is also needed to maintain the health of the epithelial tissues. Without adequate amounts of vitamin C, metabolism in these tissues probably goes slightly awry, and cancer susceptibility increases. Researchers from the Soviet Union have noticed that the vitamin C content of cervical tissue is inversely related to the degree of abnormality found in the cells: less C, more problems.

In the New York study, women with vitamin C intakes around 105 mg daily tested normal. What is absolutely staggering is that a recent national nutrition survey indicated that 35% of American women between 25 and 44 years of age consumed less than 30 mg a day! If you do not know what your typical day's intake is, then check Table 3-1. Though the RDA is 60 mg, it might be a good idea to consume double that. In looking at the chart, you can see that's easily done by several servings of fruits and vegetables daily.

You may not be able to see your cervix, but you definitely need to "C" it daily. Vitamin C is a water-soluble vitamin, meaning that excesses of it don't hang around in your body for a long time. Your best guarantee is to get some every day. There's no sense setting yourself up for a high-class Pap when you can go first class!

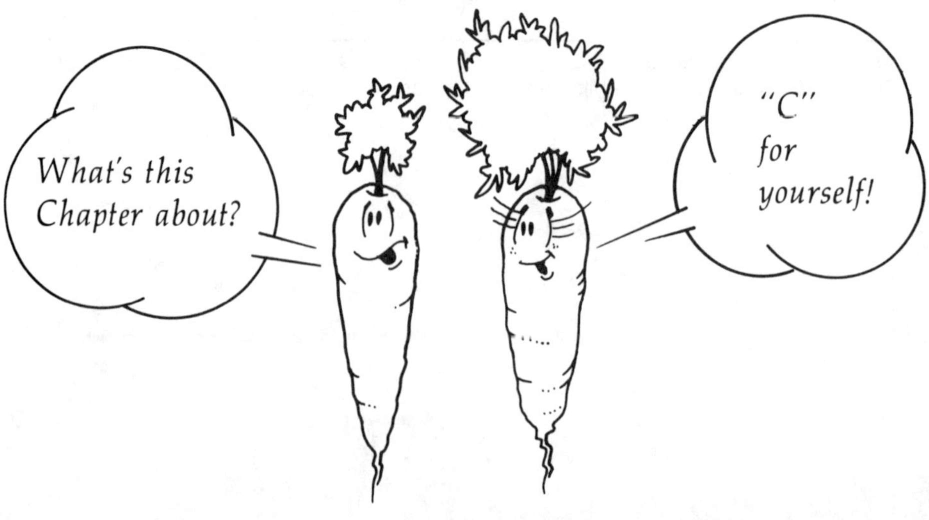

4

BIG PROSTATES

We've already discussed the prostate. However, if you're like a lot of people, you might not know where it is, let alone *what* it is or how to spell it. First of all, it's prostate, not prostrate. Men have one; women don't. The prostate is a little walnut-sized gland weighing about an ounce and situated between the bladder and rectum. The urethra passes right through it. It's in the prostate that the vas deferens, the tube that transports sperm from the testicles, hooks up with the urethra. From there the urethra heads on out through the penis and delivers either urine or sperm, depending upon what's happening at the time.

Figure 4-1: The Male Reproductive System

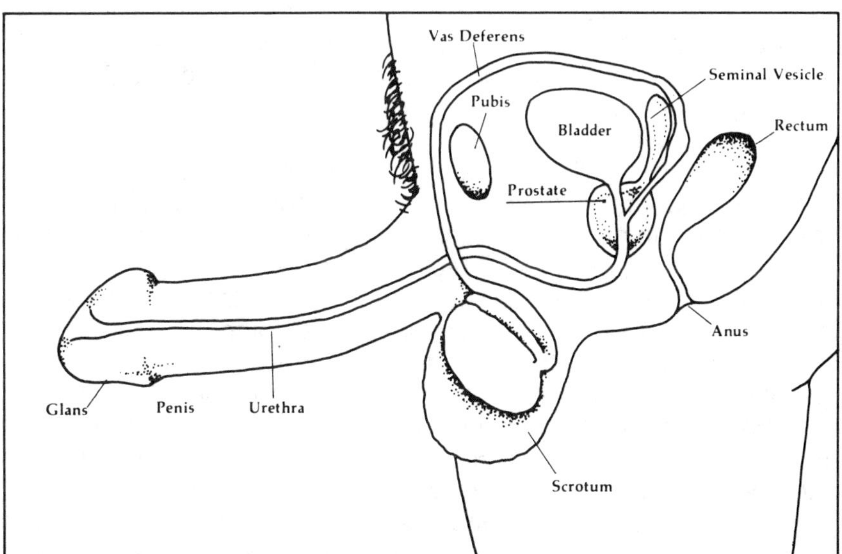

Under normal circumstances, you don't feel its presence. With a location in such a strategic place, however, a troubled prostate can make you aware that you have one. If it becomes infected or enlarged, it is likely to interfere with the simple process of taking a pee let, alone anything else. Actually, sexual intercourse can be quite uncomfortable when the prostate is enlarged.

Prostate enlargement is unlikely if you're less than 40 years old. But after that it becomes a more common occurrence with each passing decade. This condition is called "benign prostatic hypertrophy" (BPH for short). Enough to scare any set of ears, all it means is that the prostate is enlarged but not cancerous. By 50 years of age, nearly 20% of men will have BPH (too bad it's not BMW!), and the risk by 60 years of age is 50%. Needless to say, prostate trouble makes a lot of guys nervous.

Why do you have a gland that causes so much trouble? Well, the prostate has its purpose. It supplies about half of the ejaculate. Its share is rich in zinc, a mineral vital for sexual health and fertility.

When the prostate becomes enlarged, it squeezes in on the urethra and neck of the bladder. At first you hardly notice anything, except you might pee more often, have a weak stream, or a dribbly finish. You might find yourself getting up at night to go to the bathroom. Usually there's no pain. Only the condition continues to get worse. If you go to the physician (as you should for a prostate exam every six months) he can feel the prostate by inserting a gloved finger in your rectum. Though not too comfy, this kind of exam can detect BPH as well as prostate cancer, a malignancy that is the third leading cause of cancer deaths among males in the USA.

BPH starts by interfering with the urinary stream and often winds up blocking it completely. In extreme cases, this cessation of urinary flow can lead to bladder infections and kidney damage. You might say that some pee-wee problems can turn into big trouble. So rather than putting up with the associated inconvenience, see a physician and get adequate treatment.

For men with mild BPH, a few dietary changes might minimize symptoms. No matter how macho the advertisements make it look, beer will have to go. As a University of California physician wrote in the *Journal of the American Medical Association,* beer is a prostatic irritant. Why? He's not sure. It could be the hops, the malt or even the fact that you have to drink a lot of beer to get "high," and this volume of fluid might give you the sensation that you have to pee more frequently. If you don't answer the urge within a reasonable period of time, you might wind up with urinary retention, a situation bound to make your problem worse. He suggests avoiding beer completely, and keeping wine and whiskey intake to a minimum as well.

Speaking of macho, munchies laced with hot ingredients such as chili pepper and pepperoni also irritate the prostatic urethra. There is a bit of debate about the value of restricting coffee, tea and decaf. Some urologists suggest that they be taken in limited quantities or not at all. The problem with them is that they all exert a diuretic effect and can overdistend the bladder musculature, which may already be in bad shape.

If it burns when you urinate, or if you get the chills, chances are you have developed a urinary tract infection. Drinking about six to ten glasses of plain water throughout the day will cut down on bacterial growth and flush out the urethra. This may sound like a lot of water, but actually it's what is recommended for everyone. You can meet your water goal by drinking about four ounces every half hour. Then make sure you pee about every 1 1/2-2 hours. This is absolutely necessary, since you don't want to overdistend your bladder.

There doesn't appear to be any way to shrink an enlarged prostate, so treatment is usually surgical. The usual form of surgery is called a TUR (transurethral resection). This alleviates the blockage by removing the excessive tissue from the central portion of the gland while leaving the rest of it intact. Surgeons don't even have to cut to do it. Rather, they insert a special device through an anesthesized penis and take out the extra tissue, cauterizing along the way so that bleeding is kept to a minimum. The whole operation takes 45-90 minutes to complete. After a few days in the hospital it's time to go home.

With all that stuff going on down there, most men fear they will come out of the surgery with an impotence problem. But that's generally not the case. Anyone potent before the operation usually is afterwards, too. If the BPH was advanced enough to make sex uncomfortable, then the operation makes sex a lot better! You *might* be sterile—but at 50 years and above, sterility is probably a blessing, not a curse!

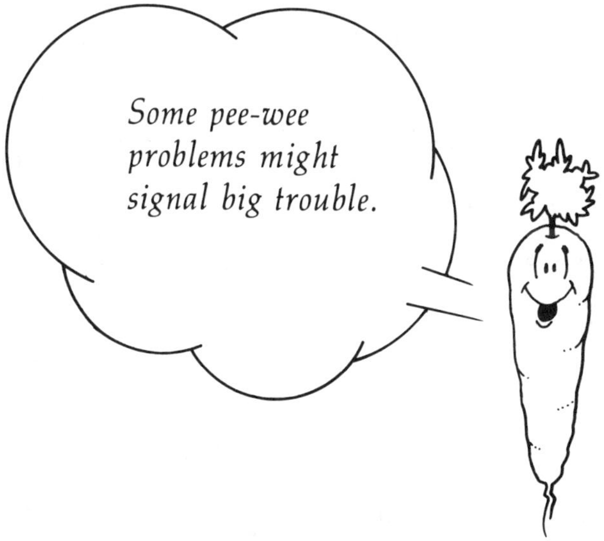

5

BIG BAD PROSTATES

When prostates are big and benign, they're troublesome. But when they're big and bad, they're cancerous. Pain "down there" is a clue. The pain can be in the penis, pelvis, rectum, back, groin and/or lower extremities. Difficulty with urination ranks high among telltale symptoms. You might think that impotence would also be a problem. It can be, but usually isn't.

Prostate cancer accounts for the majority of malignancies in men over 65 years of age. As mentioned previously, it is the third leading cause of cancer death among men in the United States, and American blacks have the world's highest death rate from prostate cancer.

At first glance, it looks like cancer of the prostate is a natural accompaniment of old age. It's a rare phenomenon in men under 40. Though few young men get it (less than 1.1% of cases occur before 50 years of age), prostate cancer is more malignant in this age group and kills more quickly. In general, as age goes up so does the incidence of prostate cancer. Survival rates show that men 50-59 years old have a higher probability of death from the disease than do older patients.

Yet age per se does not appear to be the problem. Men who have been castrated before the age of 40 never get the disease, thus indicating that hormonal factors play a role. It is also more common in the United States and in people of northern European descent. Japanese have the lowest incidence of prostate cancer, yet when they migrate to the United States and live here for 20 years or more their cancer risk begins to parallel the rest of the country. This suggests that certain environmental factors contribute to the development of prostate cancer. Among environmental factors studied, an excess amount of dietary fat appears to be a "biggie." Although researchers have discovered several pieces of the prostate cancer puzzle, they have not yet figured out how they all fit together. Let's take a look at a few of them:

One factor that pops up in medical journals is exposure to cadmium. A toxic heavy metal, cadmium has no nutritional value. In fact, you could call it anti-nutritional, because in the body it competes with zinc, a nutrient vital for prostate function. Scientists have noticed that the zinc content of cancerous prostates is one third that of healthy ones. At the same time, the cadmium content is about 25 times higher! What remains to be clarified is the old "which came first: the chicken or the egg" routine—that is, did low zinc levels precede high cadmium levels or vice versa?

Table 5-1: Some Sources of Cadmium

Environmental Sources:
Air pollution
Auto exhaust
Cigarette smoke
Electroplating industry
Industrial contamination/Incinerated industrial waste
Nickel-cadmium batteries
Plastic manufacture
Pesticides (some)

Food Sources:
Anchovies, canned
Kidney
Liver
Processing/canning of food (in some cases)
Produce grown with either superphosphate or certain organic fertilizers
Shellfish, especially oysters

Since cadmium competes with zinc, it looks as if environmental exposure to cadmium causes it to take up spots ordinarily reserved for zinc. Laboratory studies have shown that the uptake of zinc by prostatic tissue is reduced by the presence of cadmium. It just might be that a low zinc supply coupled with heavy environmental exposure makes for a potentially cancerous combo. Animal studies also suggest that this might be the case. When zinc intake is marginal, cadmium exposure causes a decrease in testicular concentration of zinc. There are no data on what goes on in prostates under these circumstances, but researchers have observed that prostate cadmium levels parallel those of testicular cadmium. So when zinc intake is low, exposure to cadmium may eventually lead to the accumulation of this toxic mineral in the prostate. This situation winds up upsetting the normal hormone-zinc balance in the prostate, a change which may lead to cancer.

Although newborns are virtually cadmium-free, cadmium accumulates with age. Getting rid of it is a slow process. Its half-life in the human body is 30 years, meaning it will take that long for half of it to disappear. Occupational exposure to cadmium dramatically heightens cancer risk. So does exposure to air pollution, but to a much lesser degree. Even so, some studies have shown that rates of prostate cancer are high in areas with a heavy concentration of suspended-particle pollution in the air. As pollution increases, deaths from prostate cancer also go up—it turns out that men living in urban areas run double the risk of those in rural parts. Poor air quality may explain, at least in part, why city dwellers are more likely to succumb to this disease. The special susceptibility of American blacks to this form of cancer is also associated with their tendency to live in cities.

Cadmium exposure is a piece of the puzzle, but not the whole picture. If it were, then there would be a lot more prostate cancer in Japan, where cadmium exposure is double that found in the USA. Here's an interesting fact for you: Japanese men have the same percentage of latent prostate cancer as American men. (A latent cancer is one which has the characteristics of a true malignancy, but lacks the capacity for growth.) This means that the Japanese have the same potential for developing prostate cancer, except that they don't get a "noticeable" disease, with symptoms, etc. It looks as though latent cancer occurs to a similar extent in many parts of the world, and variability in promotional factors in some areas apparently pushes the cancer into a full-blown, active disease.

Researchers have noted that prostate cancer is more common in men who have had more intercourse. When you think about it, every time you "do it" some zinc is lost in the ejaculate. Unless replaced by an adequate zinc intake, those zinc losses might make it easier for cadmium to settle into the prostate. (See Table 6-1 for a list of foods high in zinc!) In addition, more sex seems to be associated with more partners and a higher likelihood of venereal infection. These findings raise more questions than they answer—for instance, do sexually transmitted viruses contribute to the development of prostate cancer? Nobody knows for sure, although the possibility certainly warrants study. In the meantime, this might provide some incentive for developing a really great relationship with one woman.

All things considered, most of the research suggests that hormonal factors play a major role in the development of the "big bad prostate." And, would you believe, that's how nutrition fits into this puzzling puzzle. Here's how: Dietary fat can modify hormonal status, creating a hormonal environment within the body that appears to promote cancer growth. One striking difference between low and high-risk areas is fat intake. Areas where fat accounts for 40% of the daily caloric intake are high-risk areas. By contrast, low-risk areas are characterized by a fat intake that's only 20% of the total calories. (See

Figure 5-1). Put your right index finger on the dot for the USA. Place your left index finger on Japan's Dot. Check out the difference in fat intake. (As granny would say, "Let that be a lesson to ya.") Within the United States, prostate cancer mortality goes up as fat consumption increases. If you live in the central US, then you're in a high-risk area. Midwestern men eat lots of fat and unfortunately have the highest regional rate of prostate cancer mortality. (Too many high-fat beef meals may have really given you something to "beef" about!) Northeasterners and Westerners are next in line. Men in the Southeast have the lowest risk.

While you're reducing your fat intake, make sure you eat an ample supply of zinc. (Table 6-1) and take steps to limit your cadmium exposure (Table 5-1) as well.

Figure 5-1: Correlation between age-adjusted death rates from prostate cancer and per capita consumption of fat.

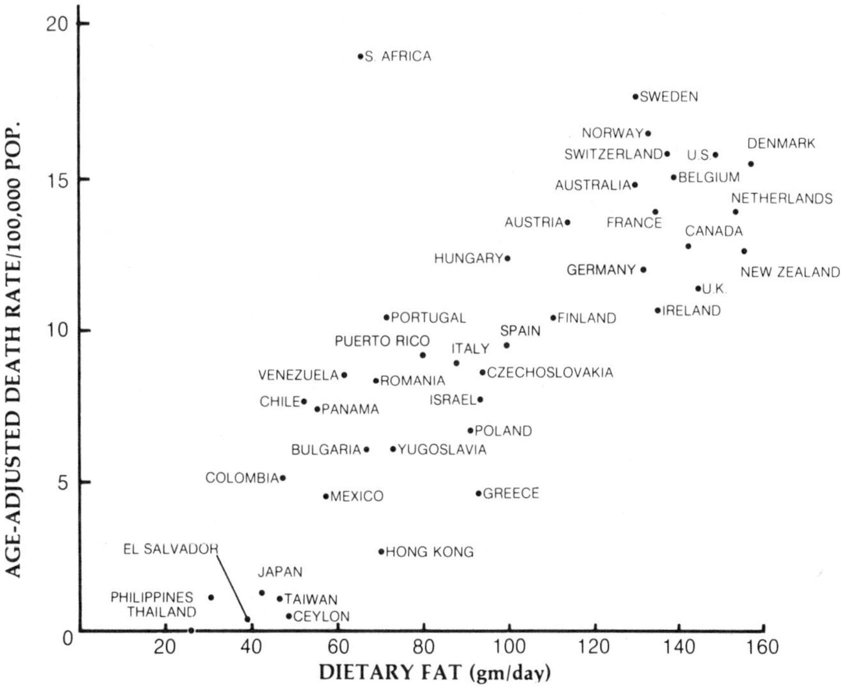

FROM: Reddy, B. S.; Cohen, L. A.; McCoy, G. D. "Nutrition and Its Relationship to Cancer," *Advances in Cancer Research*, 1980, 32.

Although this correlation is interesting, it doesn't prove that fat affects hormone status. Such a suggestive finding should not go overlooked by the scientific community, however, and it hasn't. Here's what the researchers did! They took a group of Americans (blacks and whites) eating their typical high-fat diet, and a group of South African black men, who continued to eat their usual low-fat vegetarian diet. After measuring their hormone levels while on their regular diets, they gave the Americans the vegetarian diet and the South African blacks the high-fat American diet. Urinary excretion of androgens and estrogens before the dietary switch was lower in the South Africans than in the Americans. When the diets were changed, there was an increase in the hormone excretion among the South Africans and a decrease among the Americans. Fat definitely alters hormone metabolism. Studies on laboratory animals also show that a high-fat diet changes hormone metabolism. As one researcher put it, "Any factor that affects hormonal secretion, retention, and, in particular, the sensitivity of the target organ and/or cells influences the frequency of this cancer." Since diet can modify hormonal systems, it has the potential of either enhancing or inhibiting the growth of prostate tumors. Judging from all the evidence to date, a high-fat diet appears to promote prostate cancer.

Just how zinc, cadmium, fat and hormones all interrelate is not completely understood. It will probably be a while before scientists know all the mechanics involved in prostate cancer. So where does this leave you? What can you do? One huge step toward decreasing your risk of prostate cancer would be to eat less fat. (For more details on how to go about doing that, see "Strip and Undress," Chapter 20.) Prevention-minded scientists agree that dietary intervention offers a lot of benefits, a situation where you would have little to lose and probably much to gain! Besides, being a "greaser" was never really sexy anyway!

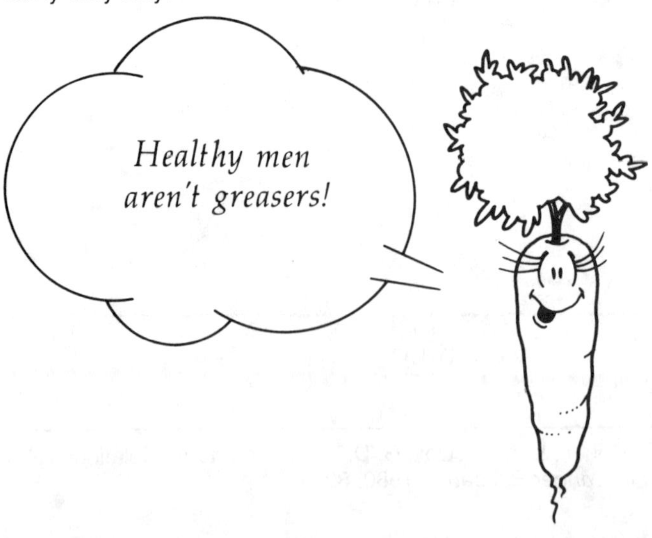

6

HOT PROSTATES

Prostates don't have to be big or bad to be sick. They can just be "hot," i.e., inflamed. The condition is called "prostatitis."

Prostatitis comes in two varieties: bacterial and abacterial. The symptoms are just about the same, except that a urinary tract infection accompanies the bacterial variety. Bacterial means there's some pathogenic (disease-causing) microbe around. The "a" on abacterial signifies there's no pathogen and rarely a problem with urinary tract infections.

So what are the symptoms of prostatitis? There are a whole bunch of them, including fever, chills and low back pain. The prostate becomes swollen and very tender. If your physician were to do a prostate exmination, he would feel an unusual warmth. There's a sense of urgency about going to the bathroom and you have to urinate frequently. This urgency and frequency have little respect for your need to sleep, so you find yourself getting up at night to go to the john. Sometimes there's even blood in your urine. There are also a lot of white blood cells in your prostatic secretions. Your prostate zinc levels go down. So does the motility of your sperm, which in turn reduces your fertility potential. (For more on sperms, see "Sperms," Chapter 7.)

While antibacterial therapy is used in bacterial prostatitis, it's obviously useless in treating the abacterial kind. Antibacterial agents are usually given for a month. This is done to prevent the development of chronic bacterial prostatitis. ("Chronic" means it will hang around with varying degrees of intensity for a long time and be a real nuisance!) Doctor Cockett, a urologist (really!), and his colleagues noticed that a month's course of antibacterials cleared up the "itis" and improved sperm motility as well. However, once the therapy was discontinued, sperm motility and prostate zinc level fell to pre-treatment levels. So they recommend that zinc therapy supplement (and/or follow) the standard treatment.

Taking zinc may also lessen the chances of a recurrence. Within the prostate there is a substance known as "prostatic antibacterial factor" which is very rich in zinc. And it looks as if the ability of this factor to kill off bacteria is related to the amount of zinc present in prostatic fluid! Researchers think that this factor may serve as a natural defense mechanism in the normal male. A decreased zinc content in the prostatic fluid may be a prelude to bacterial invasion of the prostate rather than being the effect of bacterial growth. This also means that determining the zinc content of expressed prostatic secretion may be useful in diagnosing men with chronic bacterial prostatitis and in identifying other men likely to be susceptible.

A low zinc semen level also occurs in abacterial prostatitis. Several researchers have found that supplementary zinc can boost it back to normal. To achieve this reversal in prostatic zinc status, a relatively large dose was given—between 150 and 240 mg of zinc sulfate/day. This was an effective, albeit empirical, dose. Less zinc may be as effective; future studies may shed more light on the "ideal" therapeutic dose. Will zinc also relieve the distressing symptoms of abacterial prostatitis? Some researchers have reported that doses in the 50-150 mg range can do the trick.

Taking large doses of zinc (or any metal for that matter) is not recommended for anyone who is not under medical supervision. In large doses for a relatively short period of time, zinc can be an effective form of therapy. However, large doses of zinc can also upset your stomach and produce nausea, vomiting and diarrhea. If you do use a zinc supplement, keep your total zinc (from food and supplements) below 45 mg/day.

Zinc is not only helpful in prostate diseases, it's also vital for normal sexual development. When there's not enough zinc, sex organs just don't mature. There are parts of the Middle East where hypogonadism is fairly common. The Iranian and Egyptian diet includes a lot of unleavened wheat bread, which contains phytate, a substance that binds both iron and zinc and makes them unavailable to the body. Other problems in these regions further contribute to zinc loss. (You might be wondering if hypogonadism is the Ayatollah's problem.) Impaired sexual maturity is also quite common among males with an overall reduced stature, a condition in which adolescents and young men could pass for 10-year-olds. That's because zinc is essential for growth as well as for the development of sexual organs. Interestingly, retarded growth and delayed puberty can also occur in sickle-cell anemia patients. They have excessive urinary zinc losses owing to their increased rate of red blood cell destruction.

Impotence is fairly common among men with kidney disease who are being treated by dialysis. When zinc is added to the dialysis solution, there is a striking improvement in potency and an increase in testosterone levels as well. This kind of improvement in sexual function can also occur when patients are given an oral zinc supple-

Table 6-1 Zinc Content of Food
Recommended Dietary Allowance:
15 mg
20 mg if pregnant
25 mg if breastfeeding

FOOD	SERVING SIZE	mg ZINC PER SERVING
Cereals and Grains:		
Breakfast Cereals:		
Cheerios	1 oz	0.7
Corn Flakes	1 oz	0.08
Farina, cooked	1 cup	0.2
Granola	1 oz	0.6
Millet, cooked	1 cup	1.8
Oatmeal, cooked	1 cup	1.2
Wheat bran flakes, 40%	1 oz	1.0
Wheat germ	1 tablespoon	1.7
Wheat germ, toasted	1 tablespoon	0.9
Wheat, shredded	1 oz	0.8
Wheat cereal, whole-grain, cooked	1 cup	1.2
Breads:		
Bagel	1 whole	0.5
Hamburger bun	1 whole	0.2
Italian, bread	1 slice	0.2
Pumpernickel	1 slice	0.4
Rye	1 slice	0.4
White	1 slice	0.2
Whole-wheat	1 slice	0.5
Crackers:		
Graham	2 average	0.2
Saltines	10	0.1
Whole wheat	10	0.9
Meal Accompaniments:		
Bulgur, cooked	1 cup	1.8
Noodles, soy	1 cup	2.2
Pasta, cooked	1 cup	0.7
Pasta, whole-wheat, cooked	1 cup	1.3
Rice, brown, cooked	1 cup	1.2
Rice, white, cooked	1 cup	0.8
Rice, white, instant cooked	1 cup	0.4
Fruits:		
Apple, raw	1 medium	0.8
Applesauce, unsweetened	1 cup	0.3
Apricot, dried	10 halves	0.2
Banana	1 medium	0.3
Fruit cocktail, canned	½ cup	0.02

Table 6-1 Continued (Zinc Content)

FOOD	SERVING SIZE	mg ZINC PER SERVING
Orange, raw	1 medium	.2
Peach, raw	1 medium	0.2
Pear, canned	2 halves	0.3
Raisins	2 tablespoons	.04
Strawberries	10 large	.08
Vegetables:		
Artichoke	1 medium	0.3
Avocado	½ medium	0.5
Beans, green snap	1 cup	0.4
Broccoli, cooked	1 cup	0.2
Cabbage, raw	1 cup	0.3
Cabbage, cooked	1 cup	0.6
Carrots, raw	1 medium	0.3
Carrots, boiled	1 cup	0.5
Corn, cooked	1 cup	0.7
Lettuce, head or leaf	1 cup	0.2
Onions, raw	½ cup	0.3
Peas, cooked	1 cup	1.2
Pepper, green	1	.04
Potato, baked	1 medium	1.0
Potato chips	1 oz	0.2
Spinach, raw, chopped	1 cup	0.5
Spinach, cooked	1 cup	1.3
Sprouts, bean	½ cup	0.7
Sweet Potato	1 large	0.1
Tomato, raw	1 medium	0.2
Tomato sauce	½ cup	0.7
Zucchini, cooked	1 cup	0.4
Meat, Fish, Poultry:		
Beef, lean, cooked	3 oz	4.0
Bologna	1 oz	0.5
Chicken	½ breast	0.7
	1 drumstick	1.3
Clams	3 oz	3.0
Crab	1 cup	6.7
Fish, white, fillet	3 oz	0.9
Frankfurter	1 average	0.9
Gefilte fish	3 oz	0.4
Lamb	3 oz	4.0
Liver (beef)	2 oz	3.0
Liver (chicken)	½ cup	2.3
Lobster	1 cup	3.0
Oysters, Atlantic	1 oz	25.0
Oysters, Pacific	1 oz	3.0
Pork, lean	3 oz	3.0
Scallops	3 oz	1.2
Shrimp	1 cup	2.7
Trout	3 oz	0.4
Turkey, light	3 oz	1.8
Turkey, dark	3 oz	3.7
Veal, lean	3 oz	3.5

Table 6-1 Continued (Zinc Content)

FOOD	SERVING SIZE	mg ZINC PER SERVING
Legumes (Dried Peas and Beans):		
Beans, cooked (Black, lima, pinto navy, etc.)	1 cup	1.8
Garbanzo, cooked	1 cup	2.0
Lentils, cooked	1 cup	2.0
Soy beans	1 cup	2.0
Tofu (soybean curd)	4 oz.	0.9
Nuts and Seeds:		
Almonds, roasted:	1 oz	0.7
Brazil nuts	4 nuts	0.8
Cashews	6-8	0.7
Peanuts	¼ cup	1.2
Peanut butter	2 tablespoons	1.0
Sesame seeds, raw	2 tablespoons	2.6
Sesame seeds, roasted	2 tablespoons	1.0
Sunflower seeds	2 tablespoons	0.8
Milk and Dairy Products:		
Kefir	1 cup	0.9
Milk, cow's	1 cup	1.0
Milk, goat's	1 cup	0.7
Milk, soy	1 cup	0.4
Yogurt	1 cup	1.0
Cheese:		
Cheddar	1 oz	1.0
Cottage, creamed	1 cup	1.0
Cream cheese	1 oz	.7
Most hard cheeses	1 oz	1.0
Egg	1 whole	0.5
Egg, white	1	.01
Egg, yolk	1	0.5
Miscellaneous:		
Cake, white, frosted	1 piece	.20
Chocolate bar	1 oz	.13
Cola, etc.	12 oz	.01
Cookie	1 average	.02
Danish roll	1 small	.30
Ice cream	1 cup	.60
Oil	1 tablespoon	.00
Pie (average slice)	1 piece	.02
Salad dressing	1 tablespoon	.03
Sugar	1 teaspoon	.00
Yeast (brewer's)	1 oz	2.00

Adapted from:
Freeland-Graves, J. H.; Ebangit, M. L.; Bodzy, P. W. "Zinc and Copper Content of Foods Used in Vegetarian Diets." *American Journal of Chemical Nutrition*, 1980, 77, 648-654.
Pennington, J. A.; Church, H. N. *Bowes and Church's Food Values of Portions Commonly Used.* Philadelphia: J. B. Lippincott Company, 1980.

ment to the tune of 50 mg/day. Zinc deficiency is a reversible cause of sexual dysfunction—at least in some patients with kidney failure.

As you can see, zinc is vital for your sex life. And here's a hot one for you: Zinc powers your sex drive. Too little zinc and you're in neutral. If your zinc status is OK, taking extra won't put you into "overdrive." While inadequate zinc adversely affects your sexual urge, excessive zinc will not make you the world's most "driven" lover. (Incidentally, a woman's sex drive also suffers when her zinc intake is low!)

One thing you can do for yourself is to make sure your daily zinc intake is up to snuff. Various reports indicate that a large number of people do not get the recommended daily requirement of 15 mg. Do you? Check Table 6-1 to see if today's menu dished up enough.

An adequate zinc intake is great for your love life. Consider this: Alcohol causes an increase in zinc excretion. Coffee hinders its absorption. If you tend to drink mostly booze and java, reconsider your beverage habits.

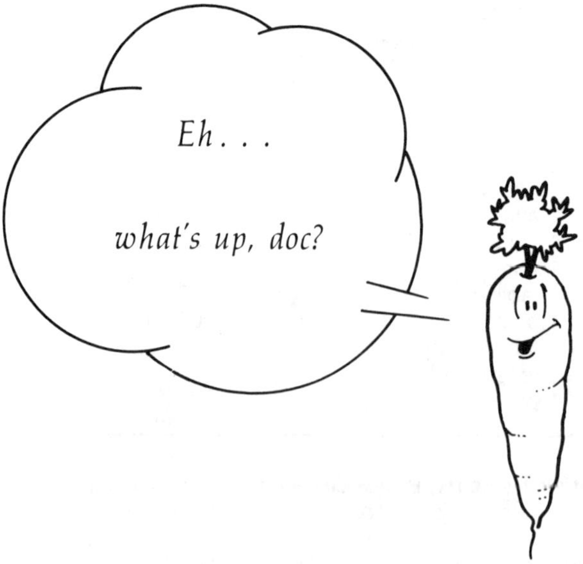

7

SPERMS

Sperms. Where would we be without them? Still a twinkle in someone's eye, no doubt. Although many nutrients are involved in the reproductive process, several play key roles in sperm production and sperm health. Among them are zinc, vitamin A and selenium.

Knowing something about sperms and sperm production will help you understand why these nutrients are vital to male fertility. Sperms originate in the seminiferous tubules in the testes; mature in the epididymous; pass through the prostate, where they really get "energized," and then head on out to their ultimate destination. How fertile you are depends, to a great degree, on how many sperms you have on your team, what kind of shape they're in and what sort of swimmers they are. (This is starting to sound like a Woody Allen movie.) Incidentally, sperm account for only about one tenth of one percent of the total semen volume.

Testicles cannot function properly without an adequate amount of vitamin A and zinc. When either is low, hormone production is altered and sperm production falls off. Even a mild zinc deficiency can adversely influence testicular function. This was demonstrated during a recent study when men were given a zinc-deficient diet. Sure enough, their sex drive decreased and their sperm count went down. An increase in dietary zinc and a low-dose zinc supplement eventually brought things back to normal.

In some cases of otherwise unexplained male infertility, low semen zinc may be the explanation. In one study researchers evaluated the fertility of a group of men. When the group's results were taken as a whole, no association could be made between zinc and fertility. So they regrouped the semen specimens into four classes according to sperm count. It turned out that each class represented a population with a different potential for fertility. Samples with the lowest zinc concentration had the lowest sperm count (less than 20 million/ml), a level considered functionally sterile. This low-zinc group also had the highest percentage of abnormal and immature sperms. In the same study another group of men with oligospermia (a sperm count less than 60 million/ml) were given zinc sulfate (80 mg three times/day) for at least six months. During that time, zinc concentration, sperm count and motility (swimming ability) all increased. Did it improve fertility? Well, nearly one fourth of the wives became pregnant during the treatment period, something that did not happen for at least an entire year before they started zinc therapy.

Anything that interferes with these nutrients may also have an effect on sperm production. That makes booze a big offender. No matter what liquor ads suggest, alcohol is anything but sexy. Alcohol competes with retinol (a form of vitamin A in the bloodstream) and, by doing so, eventually interferes with sperm production. Will one drink do it? Probably not. But one liter of whiskey (or its equivalent) per day probably will. Azoospermia (inability to produce sperm) is fairly common in chronic alcoholics. As we saw, alcohol also interferes with zinc, so it is guilty on two accounts!

In the long run, heavy-duty alcohol consumption permanently damages your testicles and liver. Since they are both involved in hormone production and balance, the ultimate effect is not a particularly happy one. It's obvious that a damaged testis will affect male sexuality. However, the liver also plays a central role in sex-hormone metabolism. Excessive alcohol can eventually "feminize" you! You become sterile and impotent. Your testicles atrophy. You lose a considerable amount of body hair. Even your breasts enlarge. This is the part about booze and sex you'll never see in liquor advertisements.

Sperm production also appears to rely on an adequate supply of B-vitamins. A deficiency impairs pituitary activity, which in turn adversely affects the testes. In short, too little male hormone is produced. An expert in the area of male infertility notes that mild B-complex deficiencies can occur during times of tension and stress. Because of that, he suggests that infertile men be given supplemental B-complex vitamins. What you eat can either bolster or jeopardize your B-vitamin status. See Table 7-1 for foods that are rich in B's. Were you aware that sugar, caffeine and alcohol rob your body of many B's?

Having sperm is not enough. They have got to be motile if they are going to compete for their job of getting the egg! It appears that sperm motility is considered one of the most important factors in the evaluation of fertility potential. The more motile the sperm, the better they swim, and good swimmers make for good fertilizers! The zinc level of the semen also parallels sperm motility. In essence, prostatic zinc "energizes" the sperm—would you believe that those spermies have got to beat their tails about ten times a second!

Other factors also affect sperm motility. Here again alcohol has an adverse effect. Eight fluid ounces of alcohol per day will not only decrease sperm production, it will also hamper sperm motility. Cigarettes impair the swim team, too: more cigarettes, less motility! The motility index in men smoking more than 30 cigarettes a day is

Table 7-1: Foods Rich in B-Vitamins

"B" HERE:	**Protein-Rich Foods:** Eggs Fish Lean meats (Pork is especially rich in thiamine) Legumes (dried peas and beans, lentils) Liver Milk Poultry Nuts **Fruits, Vegetables, Grains:** Bananas Leafy green vegetables Oatmeal Potatoes Wheat germ Whole-grain breads and cereals Yeast (brewer's)
"B" GONE SOME:	The B-Vitamins in enriched breads and cereals have only been partially restored. Unlike whole grains, they are not a good source of B-6, folic acid and pantothenic acid.
"B" GONE A LOT:	Alcohol Excessive amounts of fat and/or protein Sugar White flour products When you eat too much of these, your vitamin intake cannot keep up with your body's demand for them.

about half that of non-smokers. Also there are more deformed sperm in the semen of cigarette smokers!

Selenium is vital for spermatogenesis and motility as well: The sperm tail breaks when selenium is in short supply! (How can you swim with a broken "arm"?) So you can see why selenium is essential for fertility. It happens that in the United States, the birth rate parallels the soil selenium levels. High-selenium areas have higher birth rates. Where do you reside?

High-Selenium States:
Alabama, Arizona, Arkansas, Colorado, Iowa, Kansas, Louisiana, Mississippi, Missouri, Montana, Nebraska, Nevada, New Mexico, North Dakota, Oklahoma, South Dakota, Texas, Utah, Wyoming

Medium-Selenium States:
California, Georgia, Idaho, Kentucky, Minnesota, North Carolina, Oregon, South Carolina, Tennessee, Virginia, Washington

Low-Selenium States:
Connecticut, Delaware, Florida, Illinois, Indiana, Maine, Maryland, Massachusettes, Michigan, New Hampshire, New Jersey, New York, Ohio, Pennsylvania, Rhode Island, Vermont, West Virginia, Wisconsin, Washington, D.C.

If you're not interested in having kids and you live in a high-selenium area, don't move for fear of unwanted fertility. Instead, read on, because your testes depend on selenium too. To find out whether or not your diet supplies an adequate amount of selenium, see Table 12-1 in "Bad Breast Bumps," Chapter 12.

It's vital that you get an ample supply, because selenium protects against testicular damage caused by cadmium and possibly other environmental contaminants as well. This protective quality is related to its role as an antioxidant, i.e., an agent that protects biological tissues from hazardous interactions with oxygen and oxidants (e.g., cigarette smoke, cadmium, mercury, lead and other pollutants.) When oxidant substances combine with certain fatty acids in your body, toxic byproducts (peroxides and free radicals) are formed. Incidentally, these degradative byproducts appear to hasten the aging process and contribute to carcinogenesis! So you can see how important it is to have an adequate supply of antioxidants on your side. Other major antioxidants include vitamins C and E. Whether or not your tissues succumb to oxidant damage will depend, to a large extent, upon the strength of your antioxidant defense team and the degree of oxidative stress you encounter.

Sperm are rich in phospholipids which contain fatty acids. This makes them highly susceptible to the production of lipid peroxides, which are toxic to sperm. These harmful peroxides cause a progressive and irreversible cessation of motility and metabolic activity within the sperm. Peroxide formation also causes the sperm to become "agglutinized" (i.e., to clump together). How can a sperm swim well when it's in a huddle with its cronies? Lipid peroxidation products have been found in human sperm. Some German researchers believe that the therapeutic effect of vitamin E in the treatment of infertility can be explained by its inhibition of peroxide formation.

Vitamin C appears to be helpful in cases of infertility due to non-specific sperm agglutination. Husbands of wives who had been attempting pregnancy for two years and diagnosed as having this kind of infertility were divided into two groups. One group of twenty men were given one gram (1 gm) of viatmin C/day in a preparation

Table 7-2: Nutritional Antioxidants

VITAMIN E	Avocados, legumes, nuts, seeds, peanuts and peanut butter, vegetable oils (especially safflower oil), whole-grain breads/cereals, wheat germ. • Diets containing a lot of vegetable oils increase your need for vitamin E. Safflower oil is one of the few oils that contains an adequate ratio of vitamin E to unsaturated fat.
VITAMIN C	Broccoli, Brussels sprouts, cabbage, cauliflower, deep-green leafy vegetables, guava, sweet peppers, oranges and other citrus fruits, papaya, strawberries • For a more complete list, see Table 3-1.
SELENIUM	Asparagus, lean meats, garlic, mushrooms, organ meats (especially kidney), poultry, seafood, whole-grain breads and cereals, yeast grown on selenium-rich soil • For a complete list, see Table 12-1. • A 50-150 mcg supplement has been recommended for vegetarians.

that also contained calcium, manganese and magnesium. The therapy period lasted sixty days. Another group of seven men did not get therapy. All the wives of the men receiving the supplement became pregnant during the study period while the other wives did not. When semen samples of the men were examined under a microscope, the "sperm clumps" universally present prior to the study were not present in the samples from men who had received the supplementation. The vitamin C level of the semen in supplemented subjects tripled. Sperm motility also increased in this group. Because previous studies have demonstrated the ability of vitamin C to reverse sperm agglutination, these researchers believe that vitamin C can bring about dramatic improvements in this form of infertility. However, they also acknowledge that the supplemented minerals may have contributed as well.

When sperm are subjected to oxidant stress, they quit swimming. When your testes are exposed (to oxidant stress, that is), not only does sperm production decrease, but your risk of testicular cancer goes up.

During the last 30 years, the average sperm density in the USA has declined appreciably. From 1929 to 1951, sperm density averaged 100-145 million/ml. By 1970 it had dropped to 48-80 million/ml.

Several factors have been suggested as potential causes, including tight-fitting underpants, an increased frequency of ejaculation and an increased exposure to toxic substances. Tight-fitting underwear is suspected because it holds the testes very close to the body. As a result, they might get warmer than they're supposed to be. (They hang outside because they need to be several degrees cooler than body temperature for sperm production to proceed normally.) Excessive ejaculation (several times a day for ten or more days) may be the culprit because demand exceeds sperm production capabilities. But "hot balls" and "hot times" may not be the major reasons. That leaves environmental contamination. And that's serious, because it may put homo sapiens on the endangered species list!

Studies at Florida State University have found toxic chemicals in semen samples from student volunteers. Several of these chemicals are known carcinogens or teratogens (substances causing birth defects). The sperm counts of the students averaged only 20 million/ml. Nearly one fourth of the students were classified as functionally sterile! There's more evidence: Workers producing chlorinated hyprocarbon pesticides report they cannot conceive children; Vietnam vets exposed to Agent Orange have high rates of birth defects among their children. Usually birth defects are associated with the mother. That the male can contribute to deformities is a relatively recent finding.

During the same time that sperm counts are decreasing, testicular cancer rates are going up—especially in young men. A hundred years ago, most of the men with testicular cancer were elderly. By the 1950s, 12% of the cases were in men under 25 years of age. Today that has doubled: 25% of men with testicular cancer are under 25! The testicles are very sensitive to environmental toxins. A doctor at the National Institute of Occupational Safety and Health even suggests that testing the sperm counts of workers would be helpful in monitoring the safety of industrial chemicals.

The decline of the Roman Empire has been blamed on many things, lead poisoning among them because it could have caused infertility in the male subjects. In the USA today lead has even been reported in the semen of healthy men who were not considered victims of lead poisoning! There's plenty of lead in urban environments: Is this why testicular cancer has tripled in blacks since the 1950s? Has their cancer rate followed their migration to the cities?

For your own protection, (a) decrease your exposure to environmental pollution as much as possible, (b) wash fruits and vegetables thoroughly to remove pesticide residue, and (c) eat lots of wholesome foods. Make sure you include foods rich in selenium, vitamins A, E, and C and zinc. I'd get a copy of the American Cancer Society's brochure on testicular self-exam and check myself out as it suggests. By the way, I'd call my physician pronto if I found anything abnormal.

Sperms are so little, yet I've written a lot about them. For one thing, I found them very interesting! However, I'm also concerned about our national sperm crisis. You might be thinking it's no big deal. After all, there are too many people these days anyway. But I look at it this way: Choosing not to have children when you can is one thing. Wanting a child and not being able to have one is very different—especially if the reason is environmentally-induced. Keep yourself well-nourished. Environmental pollution and other forms of oxidative stress are more hazardous to a body that's inadequately nourished with vitamins C and E and selenium.

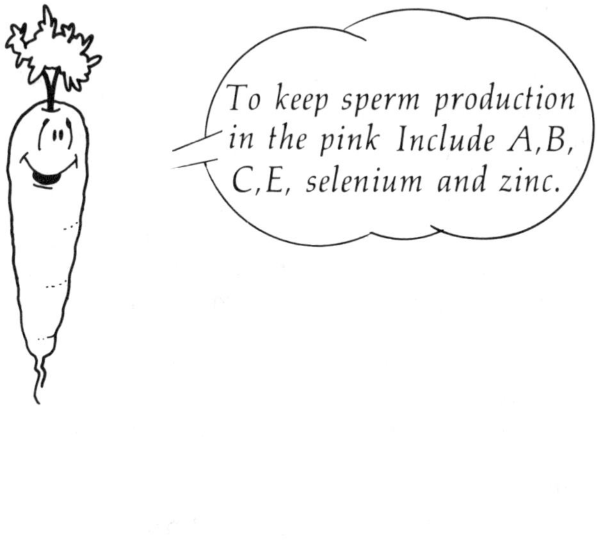
To keep sperm production in the pink Include A,B, C,E, selenium and zinc.

8

THE PILL

Here I've gone on about how to keep those sperm healthy and in the swim. But what happens when you don't want the swimmers to get to the goal? Remember that old chestnut about the best birth control pill? (An aspirin in between your knees! It works, but it doesn't do much for your love life.) What about "The Pill"? When used properly, oral contraceptives make birth control a snap, but they are not without their own problems. Recently there have been warnings about an increased risk of skin cancer among pill users, and it's been known for years that women who smoke and use the pill have a high risk of blood clots, heart disease and strokes. This is the newsworthy stuff, and you probably know it already.

If you have taken birth control pills, you probably also know that they can make you feel depressed. One of the reasons for this is that the pill interferes with normal pyridoxine (vitamin B-6) metabolism. This can contribute to anxiety and depression in up to 40% of the women on the pill. One study of depressed oral contraceptive users showed that a supplement of 40 mg of pyridoxine hydrochloride improved the depression and other indices of B-6 deficiency. The supplement was not helpful in depressed women who were not B-6 deficient. Here's something else to make you feel more depressed: The vitamin B-6 deficiency can lead to a decrease in the ol' libido! That's a curious side effect for a "liberating" pill!

Whether or not all women on the pill need supplementary B-6 is still questionable at this time. Women who develop depression during pill use may benefit from a dose as high as 40 mg. (Note: The RDA is only 2.0 mg.) However, if supplementation were started as soon as contraceptive use began, then a much lower dose would probably be helpful in avoiding problems associated with B-6 deficiency. A daily intake of 5 mg appears adequate to meet the needs of most oral contraceptive users.

About 10% of pill users wind up with a disturbance in glucose tolerance. This is especially true in women with a past history of abnormal glucose metabolism, a family history of diabetes, delivery of an excessively large infant, obesity or excessive weight gain. This impairment of glucose metabolism in many women appears to be associated with B-6 deficiency and can be relieved with supplements containing two-to-three times the RDA taken daily while on the pill. If you choose to go off the pill, the abnormalities in glucose tolerance will reverse within three months after discontinuing its use.

A deficiency of B-6 can interfere with your sex life, because it is associated with a strong tendency to develop infections, particularly of the genito-urinary tract. An infection "down there" can put you out of commission for a while. Actually, an infection anywhere may dampen the urge and/or the ability to follow through. Vitamin B-6 is one of many nutrients required by the immune system, so make sure you get your fair share.

If you have a passion for white bread and sweets you'll have trouble getting an adequate supply of B-6, even if you're not taking the pill. Superimposing the pill on a lousy diet makes depression more likely, but including foods rich in B-6 will help. The best sources are: whole-grain breads and cereals, lean meat, liver, potatoes and sweet potatoes, dark-green leafy vegetables, egg yolk, fish and shellfish, legumes, peanuts and peanut butter, walnuts, filberts, prunes and raisins and brewer's yeast. Canning and freezing causes extensive loss of B-6 from vegetables. So does the canning of meat and fish. Ninety percent of the B-6 is milled out of white flour; none is added back into the "enriched" (i.e., impoverished) white bread. Go easy on the protein foods—a very high protein diet can hasten the onset of a deficiency! How much protein do you really need? See Table 9-1.

Other vitamins are also affected by oral contraceptive use. The pill seems to deteriorate thiamine status. Supplements of 3 mg/day of thiamine (B-1) prevent some of the biochemical disruptions caused by use of the pill. Considering that thiamine is "the morale vitamin," and essential for a healthy outlook, make sure you're well supplied. Whole-grain and enriched breads and cereals, liver, pork, fish, lean meat, poultry, milk, legumes and some fresh vegetables are your best sources. However, you should know that sugar, alcohol and caffeine also increase your demand for it without supplying any! Too much of them further jeopardizes your thiamine status. When thiamine is low relative to your actual needs you can feel depressed, irritable, tired and apathetic—not exactly the characteristics of a femme fatale.

There may also be problems with riboflavin (B-2). Use of the pill aggravates any pre-existing deficiency. As mentioned previously, riboflavin deficiency is not that uncommon in the U.S. Studies have shown a correlation between milk intake, a wholesome diet and riboflavin status. This means that anyone who has difficulties with milk (e.g., lactose deficiency, which is common in blacks) may need a little extra ribo-boost. A supplement containing 2.0 mg/day seems to do the trick for women whose riboflavin status is already poor before starting on the pill.

It appears that pill users would benefit from a little extra vitamin C as well. Many women on oral contraceptives have been found to have low blood levels of this vitamin. In studying the effect of oral contraceptives on vitamin C, researchers provided 155 mg/day to women on and off the pill. No difference was found between users and non-users. However, 155 mg is two and a half times higher than the RDA. Perhaps this generous amount is enough to guard against the low blood levels of vitamin C that do develop in women on the "pill." It's pretty easy to eat 155 mg/day. (See Table 3-1 in "High-Class Pap," Chapter 3, to find out how much you usually eat.)

While blood levels of the B-complex and vitamin C go down, that of vitamin A goes up. That looks promising, but it isn't. The blood level goes up because more of the vitamin is being pulled out of storage from the liver. For someone who's not into carrots, etc., this is not great news, because the pill could cause a gradual depletion of your liver stores of vitamin A. So vitamin A requirements are increased by the pill. There's no need to run out and get huge amounts of the stuff. One researcher suggests a supplement containing 5,000 IU. Given an RDA of 5,000 IU, that may mean doubling the requirement. It's easy to get that increased amount from food. However, it takes more than one small carrot. You'd better go back to Table 1-1 in "Sex and the Single Carrot," Chapter 1. Or else just eat one helluva carrot every day!

Studies repeatedly show that women on the pill have low blood levels of folic acid. This can be normalized by folic acid supplementation during use of the pill. Supplementation may also reverse another abnormality associated with disturbed folic acid metabolism: enlarged cervical and vaginal cells, This abnormality was corrected when women were given 100 mg of folic acid daily during the time they used contraceptive pills.

A recent report has also shown that folic acid supplementation may reduce the risk of cervical cancer in women taking oral contraceptives. There is no strong evidence showing that the pill increases risk of cervical cancer. However, in women who have cervical dysplasia (tissue abnormality), the pill seems to hasten the change from dysplasia to cancer. In this recent study, young women on birth control pills who had mild to moderate cervical dysplasia were divided into two groups. One received a "therapeutic" dose (10 mg) of folic acid each day for three months, while the others got a placebo. The folate supplementation had a substantial benefit on the cervical tissue. The researchers found that the dysplasia disappeared in several women taking folic acid. In other women, the supplement seemed to reduce its progression. Cancer did not develop in any of the women in the folic acid group. However, several women in the placebo group showed signs of early, possibly precancerous, changes. It is not certain that the form of dysplasia found ("cervical intraepithelial neoplasia") is actually a precancerous lesion. But if it is, then additional folic acid may help reduce cancer risk in women who take the pill and who also have cervical dysplasia. (For more on cervical cancer, see "High-Class Pap," Chapter 3.)

The folic acid requirement for women on the pill is higher than that for non-users. Interestingly, folic acid deficiency is the most common form of vitamin deficiency, and is easily brought about by avoidance of folate-rich foods. If you skip fresh produce, then your diet might be low. (See Table 8-1 for foods high in folate.) Birth control pills can precipitate a deficiency if you neglect these foods!

Table 8-1: Foods Full of Folic Acid

Asparagus
Beet greens
Bok choy
Brussels sprouts
Cabbage
Chard
Cilantro
Green leafy vegetables (Hint: foliage for folate!)
Legumes
Liver
Mint
Nuts
Oranges
Parsley
Red leaf lettuce
Romaine
Scallions
Spinach
Watercress
Whole-wheat products
Yeast (brewer's)

FOLATE FACTS

Heating or processing at high temperatures causes large losses. Normal cooking temperatures (110-120°C) for ten minutes can cause losses up to 65%. Nearly 70% of it is lost if vegetables are stored at room temperature for three days., Folic acid is not usually added to fortified or enriched foods.

Incidentally, some women run a high risk of having a nutritional problem when they use the pill! What about you?

— Have you just had a baby?
— Are you planning to have one soon after getting off the pill?
— Have you recently been sick or had surgery?
— Do you have poor eating habits?
— Are you dieting all the time? Anorexic? Bulemic?
— Are you a teenager?

If you fit into one or several of these categories, chances are your nutritional status is not up to snuff. If you intend to become pregnant soon after going off the pill, any deficiency you've had before will become worse. Pregnancy places a set of its own nutritional demands on you. Malnourished women have a higher risk of having babies that are smaller than the average newborn and/or have birth defects. Even if you are not planning on having a child soon, it's still important that you eat well.

Here's a little supplementary advice: To get the additional increment in vitamin intake, don't go out and buy a bunch of bottles, each containing a different vitamin! A relatively low-dose, broad-spectrum multivitamin/mineral formula will probably fill in the gap between a good diet and the increased nutritional demands brought on by the pill. Get one that includes the dosage recommendations just discussed. Also make sure that it contains folic acid (some don't). Since you'll be eating foods that contain folate, you will not need a supplement that contains any more than 400 mcg.

Now that you're on the pill, there's a special urgency to get fresh every day (fresh fruits and vegetables, that is!).

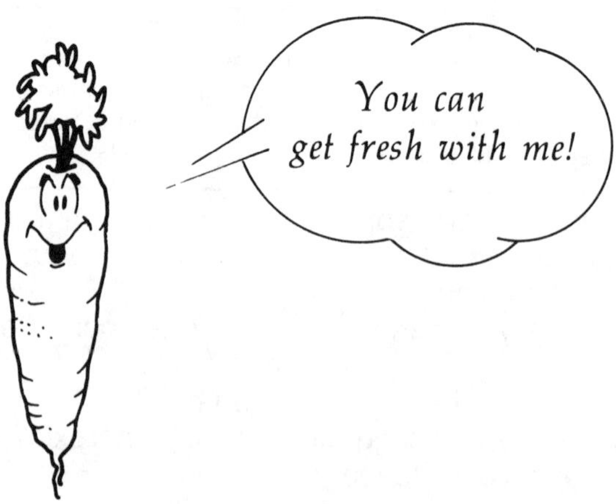

9

THE CURSE

It's getting to be "that time of the month." Do you feel irritable, bloated, depressed and/or have a craving for sweets? If you do during the 7-14 days before you have your period, but not when you have it, then chances are you have "premenstrual tension syndrome," PMT for short. It's also called premenstrual syndrome (PMS).

PMS has been called other things, including the melancholies of menstruation, premenstrual water toxemia, and menstrual psychosis, even "the witch syndrome." Some people do not believe that PMS exists. These are the people who tell you "it's all in your head"! Well, PMS is a very real experience for nearly half of all menstruating women, and it's most likely to affect women between the ages of 31-40. PMS tends to get progressively worse as women get older and have more pregnancies. As many as 40% of women with these premenstrual changes are substantially disturbed by them. Another 20% are seriously disabled because of them.

The mood swings and behavior changes that accompany PMS are often severe enough to disturb family relationships. Several years ago in England, the premenstrual syndrome was established as a mitigating condition in women who commit serious crimes.

Conventional therapies for PMS include hormones, aspirin, diurectics, sedatives, tranquilizers and narcotics. Unfortunately, these tend to treat the symptoms, not the underlying cause, and they are often ineffective. A handful of physicians in the U.S. and England have been exploring nutritional approaches that appear very promising.

A leader in the nutritional treatment of PMS and former professor of OB-GYN at the UCLA School of Medicine, Doctor Guy Abraham, has found that premenstrual tension symptoms can be clustered into four distinct groups. You might fit into one or several categories.

PMS-A
This is the most common one, with nearly 80% of all PMS patients having these symptoms: anxiety, irritability, nervous tension and mood swings. If you have this, you'll start having symptoms as early as two weeks before your period. You feel progressively worse, sometimes even depressed (which is PMS-D), until you get your period. Then you feel better.
PMS-H
PMS-H is also popular, just a little less so than the "A" variety. About 60% of women with PMS complain of PMS-H symptoms, among them a sensation of weight gain during the few days right before your period. You've got that bloated feeling; your breasts feel tender. You also probably notice some swelling in your face, hands and feet. You might feel like you gained a ton, but most women gain less than three pounds. A few gain as much as 20 pounds! This weight gain can be a problem. As age increases, not all the weight is lost during menstruation. So every month, a bit more weight hangs on.
PMS-C
About 40% of PMS sufferers have this kind. This is when your appetite increases before your periods. You crave sweets (mainly chocolates), especially if you're under stress. So you eat a lot of sweets, and a few hours later you're fatigued and headachey. Your heart pounds. You feel like fainting. You might even get "the shakes."
PMS-D
Occurring less frequently than the other varieties. PMS-D is when you feel depressed, withdrawn, confused and forgetful before your periods. You might find yourself crying easily and you might have difficulty sleeping. Most women with this type also have PMS-A. In this combination your nervousness and irritability give way to depression and other symptoms a few days before you get your period. It's much less common to have PMS-D all by itself.

However, when it does occur alone women can actually feel suicidal. They also feel lethargic, incoherent and have difficulty verbalizing. This is a serious situation and needs medical attention. For some odd reason, most women with PMS-D (unaccompanied by PMS-A) don't seek out help for themselves; it's usually a friend or relative who brings them to a psychiatrist.

What's behind all these uncomfortable and distressing symptoms? The premenstrual tension syndromes involve a complex interplay of hormone balance, stress and nutritional deficiencies (involving especially the B-complex vitamins and magnesium.) In determining the "why" of it all, Doctor Abraham suggests a different chain of causal events for each type of PMS, with nutritional factors playing a significant role each time.

Even as early as 1943, supplemental B-vitamins were shown to have a positive effect on PMS patients. Since then researchers have discovered that very high doses of B-6 reduce the severity of PMS symptoms, including a decrease in premenstrual "bloat." Meanwhile, the women taking B-6 noticed they felt less tense, less anxious and were better able to cope. They also slept better throughout the night and had higher energy levels during the day. Their menstrual cramps were less severe. In some women, the cramps completely disappeared. (For more on cramps, see "The Cramps," Chapter 10.) A number of women with a previous history of unexplained infertility conceived. The researchers suggest that B-6 therapy may be rewarding in infertile PMS patients who have had difficulty getting pregnant.

Magnesium deficiency has been found to be commonplace among women with PMS. Here's another interesting fact about magnesium. During stressful situations, magnesium excretion is increased. PMS can be triggered by stress. Since PMS itself is stressful, it might cause further magnesium depletion! It appears that many of the PMS symptoms can be explained on the basis of magnesium deficiency, so it's been suggested that red cell magnesium determinations be included by physicians in their evaluation of PMS. One reason why B-6 therapy is helpful may be related to its role in helping to transport magnesium into the cells.

If you found that one or several types of PMS describes your experience of premenstrual melancholia, here are a few suggestions for you. First of all, learn how to deal with stress, since it worsens PMS. So does the lack of outdoor physical activity. Take yourself out each day and you'll kill two birds with one stone—exercise is a great stress reducer! Get walking shoes and/or a dog. When you have to take the dog out, you'll find you no longer have any excuse not to exercise. You'll be in deep doggy #@!* if you don't! Walk briskly for several miles each day. Do it with the dog, a friend, a walking club, a spouse, a lover. Or else just go alone and enjoy the time to yourself.

You also need to make sure that your diet favors a positive balance of B-vitamins and magnesium. So include foods that are rich in both: whole grains, green leafy vegetables, and legumes. Sugar increases your need for B-vitamins and magnesium. Alcohol does too, since it increases their excretion. You'd do well to restrict sweets and spirits. Keep your sugar intake below two tablespoons a day. Would you believe—a 12-oz. soda contains three! (See "Getting Stoned," Chapter 15, for more on sugar.) Have no more than one ounce of alcohol per day. You'll find an ounce of alcohol in two jiggers of hard liquor, or two 12-oz. cans of beer, or one 6- to 8-oz. glass of wine. Caffeine also increases your body's need for B-vitamins. So it's a good idea to limit your caffeine intake (For more on caffeine, see "Breast Bumps," Chapter 11.)

In studying the dietary differences of women with and without PMS, the researchers found that PMS patients had relatively poor eating habits. PMS patients ate fewer whole grains and other high-fiber foods, more protein and a relatively large amount of dairy products. They were also eating almost seven tablespoons of sugar per day, while women without PMS averaged two tablespoons daily.

Interestingly, certain foods, if eaten excessively, can interfere with magnesium retention and absorption. This includes protein, fat and dairy products. Now don't go exclude them completely. Rather, keep your intake in line with your actual requirements. This is pretty easy to do. Here are some guidelines:

#1 See Table 9-1 to determine how much protein you really do need.
#2 Have no more than two servings of milk, yogurt or cheese daily. How much is a serving? See Table 14-1.
#3 Cut down on your fat consumption, too. See "Strip and Undress," Chapter 20, for more information on fat.
#4 Include a tiny bit of essential fat (linoleic acid) daily. Vegetable oils are good sources, provided they have not been hydrogenated. So beware of margarines and solid vegetable shortenings. Liquid safflower oil is your best bet. Use a little in your salad dressing and when sautéing.

Incidentally, cutting back on salty stuff will also help dispel the curse of premenstrual bloat. (See "Passion and Potency," Chapter 22, for more information on salt.)

In their own special program for PMS, the researchers are using a uniquely formulated multivitamin/mineral supplement that contains some magnesium and a generous amount of B-6. This has been found be be effective in managing PMS, especially when combined with the previously-outlined dietary improvements and some regular exercise.

There's been a big discussion of B-6 and magnesium. Whatever you do, do not go out and buy a supplement bottle of each. It's not a good idea to take nutrients separately, since an excess of one nutrient may adversely affect the others. If you're plagued by PMS, improve your diet and exercise habits. (For more information about PMS and an appropriate supplementation program to accompany the suggested changes in dietary habits, check out the "Resources" section.)

Meanwhile in Britain, some more exciting nutritional research is going on. Physicians at the St. Thomas Hospital Medical School have

Table 9-1: Protein Content of Foods

The recommended amount of protein is smaller than you think. The average woman needs only 44 grams a day and the average man, 56 grams. Certain situations increase protein requirements (e.g., surgery, illness.) Some preliminary studies indicate that "seniors" may need more than the younger set.

Figure 0.8 to 1.0 gram of protein for every 2.2 pounds you weigh.

Your weight ________ lbs. divided by 2.2 = ________ × 0.8 (or 1) = ________ gms/day.

Pregnant? Add 30 gm/day.
Breast feeding? Add 20 gm/day.

FOOD	SERVING	AVERAGE PROTEIN/SERVING
Protein Foods of Animal Origin:		
Meat	1 oz	7
Fish	1 oz	7
Poultry	1 oz	7
Egg	1	7
Milk	8 oz	8
Cheese, cheddar-type	1 oz	7
Cheese, cottage	½ cup	15
Yogurt, lowfat	1 cup	12
Yogurt, whole	1 cup	8
Protein Foods of Plant Origin:		
Beans, cooked	½ cup	8
Soybeans, cooked	½ cup	11
Soybean curd (tofu)	3½ oz	8
Soybean milk	1 cup	9
Nuts	1 oz	5
Seeds, pumpkin	1 oz	8
Seeds, sesame	1 oz	5
Other Foods:		
Grains:		
Bagel	1	6
Biscuit	1	2
Bread, white	1 slice	2
Bread, whole-grain	1 slice	3
Cereals, cold	1 oz	2
Cereals, whole-grain, cooked	½ cup	3
Muffin	1 average	3
Pancake	1 average	3
Pasta, cooked (spaghetti, noodles)	1 cup	7
Rice, white, cooked	1 cup	3
Tortilla	1 6" diam	2
What germ, toasted	¼ cup	9

Table 9-1 Continued (Protein content)

FOOD	SERVING	AVERAGE PROTEIN/SERVING
Vegetables:		
Broccoli	1 5" stalk	4
Greens (collards)	1 cup, cooked	7
Greens (spinach, kale)	1 cup, cooked	5
Mushrooms	10 small	3
Potato	1 medium	2
Vegetables not listed	½ cup	1-2 (average)
Fruits:		
Average piece		½-1

Even just by glancing at the chart, you can see how easy it is to meet your protein requirements, whether you're a meat-eater or vegetarian!

been experimenting with the use of evening primrose oil as a treatment for PMS. More than 70 women with severe PMS, who found no relief with the more traditional therapies, were given supplements of evening primrose oil, an oil that is a uniquely rich source of essential fatty acids. A large percentage (67%) of the women had complete relief of symptoms; another 22% had partial relief! There were very few side effects. Three patients had skin blemishes; three others had transient mood changes.

What's so special about this oil? Evening primrose oil contains a fatty acid that is not found in many foods, with the exception of human milk. This particular fatty acid, gamma linoleic acid (GLA), can also be made in your body from linoleic acid. Several nutrients are required for its production, including magnesium. GLA is a precursor of yet another substance that's made in your body, prostaglandin E-1.

Prostaglandins are involved in the step-by-step regulation of many functions within the body. To date, about 30 prostaglandins have been identified, each with a specific range of action. Some of them have highly favorable effects while others exert less favorable ones. Prostaglandin E-1 (PGE-1) is among those with positive effects. If the formation of GLA is reduced, then the production of PGE-1 falls off. PMS may be related to problems in producing this prostaglandin.

Several nutrients are necessary for PGE-1 production, including B-6, magnesium, zinc, B-3 (niacin) and vitamin C in addition to linoleic acid. If any are missing, then the process cannot be completed, and your body does not get the beneficial effect of the prostaglandin. As mentioned previously, many women with PMS are deficient in magnesium. The excessive amount of sugar and refined foods they eat can also bring on a deficiency of B-6. In addition, many young women have been found to have diets low in zinc, because of a limited calorie intake and poor food choices as well. As mentioned previously, an inadequate intake of vitamin C is not that uncommon, either! Though the use of vegetable oil has increased, most is hydrogenated. During the hydrogenation process, much (if not all) of the linoleic acid is destroyed. That's why a diet chock full of processed vegetable oils will hamper PGE-1 production, and so will an excessive amount of animal fats and alcohol. Just in case you haven't seen the similarities: The dietary improvements outlined previously favor the formation of this "friendly" prostaglandin.

The nutritional approach to PMS is exciting, albeit relatively new and probably not tested as much as some medical people would prefer. There is still a lot to be learned about PMS. Since many women have benefited from nutritional therapy, the outlook for the future looks a lot brighter. Think about your typical eating style. If it needs some sprucing up, then do it.

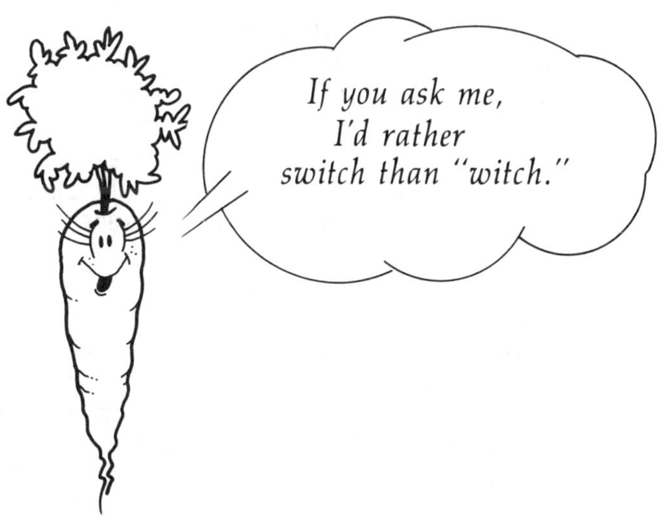

10
THE CRAMPS

Painful periods and premenstrual tension are two different things. Premenstrual tension is what goes on before you get your period. Cramps are what you might feel when you have it. In medical lingo, cramps are called dysmenorrhea. Women who have PMT often get menstrual cramps, too. These cramps are most intense immediately before or upon starting your period.

Dysmenorrhea comes in two varieties, primary and secondary. The secondary type is usually associated with a demonstrable cause, such as endometriosis, a tumor or another tangible problem. Until recently the primary variety was little understood, albeit "popular," with incidence rates running as high as 40% or more. It begins in adolescence when ovulation first begins. It tends to diminish over time, unlike PMS, which worsens with age. In addition, regular sexual intercourse and pregnancy help dispel these painful cramps.

Hormonal imbalances and psychogenic factors (i.e., "it's all in your head") are believed to be part of the picture. However, current research suggests it's the excessive production of certain prostaglandins that put the cramp in your style.

As mentioned previously, prostaglandins are regulatory substances that are manufactured in your body. In the uterus there are two major prostaglandins, E and F, which regulate uterine contractions. Prostaglandin F stimulates the intensity and frequency of contractions, whereas prostaglandin E relaxes the uterine muscles. Throughout the menstrual cycle, prostaglandin E levels remain constant, while synthesis of the F variety is increased during the latter half. Maximum release of prostaglandins occurs during menstruation.

This discovery of the relationship of prostaglandins to menstrual cramps has prompted the use of new drugs, prostaglandin inhibitors. These are among the most common forms of therapy for severe cramps, and are much more effective than aspirin. Reported results with prostaglandin inhibitors show that they can be dramatically successful in bringing relief. Like most drugs, though, they are not without side effects: Headaches, drowsiness, stomach trouble, vomiting, diarrhea, dizziness and skin rash are occasionally observed in patients using them.

Dysmenorrhea has not escaped the queries of nutrition researchers either. Magnesium relaxes the uterine muscle, and magnesium deficiency has been implicated as the cause of dysmenorrhea. Subsequent studies have discovered low tissue magnesium levels in women with this problem. During a study of women with dysmenorrhea, combined B-6 and magnesium therapy was given. (Remember? B-6 helps transport magnesium into the cell.) Not only was there a significant improvement in symptoms, but tissue magnesium levels increased also. However, it took about four to six months for this therapy to reach its maximum effectiveness. During the early course of nutritional therapy, the researchers did recommend the use of prostaglandin inhibitors to quell the early discomfort.

If your monthly cramp crimps your style, take the time to evaluate your eating habits. You might not be getting an adequate magnesium supply. (See preceding chapter, "The Curse," for more information on magnesium.) A nutritional program similar to what's described there also appears to benefit some women with menstrual cramps. It might even help with irregular periods.

Menstrual regularity depends on a variety of factors, and several are related to nutrition. For instance, the onset of menstruation in young women is dependent on attaining a critical body weight and/or body fat. You have undoubtedly heard that women with unusually low percentages of body fat, such as ballet dancers and extremely athletic women, quit having their periods. It's also been shown that fasting and excessive weight loss can inhibit monthly cycles and ovulation. Refeeding can reinitiate them.

Extreme dietary restriction is not the only dietary alteration that changes hormonal activity. Women eating a lot of refined foods have different hormonal patterns than do women eating "whole" unrefined foods. When a high-fat, high-sugar diet that's also high in animal protein is given to a woman whose usual diet is essentially low in fat and high in unrefined plant foods, her hormonal patterns change. This was seen recently when rural black South African premenopausal women were given a typical American diet. During the time of the feeding study, their hormone profiles did not remain constant. Instead, they began to resemble those found in American women with menstrual abnormalities!

Being fat also interferes with normal hormonal activity. Obese women tend to have cycles of irregular lengths, with the average cycle being more than 36 days long. It's also common for them to have heavy menstrual flows, and to go through a cycle without ovulating.

Although all the delicate relationships between diet, body fat and hormones are not totally understood, the evidence indicates that poor diets disrupt normal hormonal relationships, which can lead to painful or irregular periods and, by interfering with ovulation, hamper fertility. So bad diets may sentence you to problematical periods.

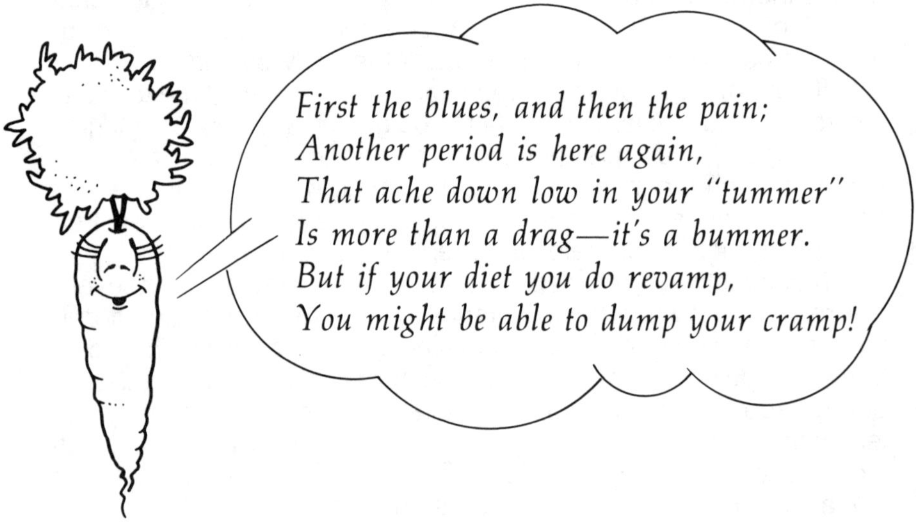

11

BREAST BUMPS

Do you have lumpy, painful breasts? If you are like a lot of premenopausal women, you do. In medical jargon lumpy, painful breasts are referred to as fibrocystic breast disease, the most common female breast disorder around. Recently there has been some debate as to whether it's a "disease" or a normal variation. Whatever you call it, it's a benign (non-cancerous) condition. However, women with cystic breasts may run a higher risk of developing breast cancer than women who have never had the condition.

How do you know if you've got it? If you are bothered by breast pain (especially before and during your period), you probably do. If you don't have any pain, then give yourself a breast exam. If you find that one or both of your breasts have a lumpy nodular consistency, it would be a good idea to have the situation checked out by a physician. The problem with these lumps is that they can camouflage cancerous tissue. This may give your physician a tough time in discerning the nature of your problem. When this is the case, additional tests can be ordered to confirm that your problem is benign. (Incidentally, if you do have cystic breasts, it's a smart idea to stop by your physician's office every six months for a check up.)

Until recently there has been no effective therapy for relieving the discomfort of cystic breasts, leaving you with two choices: 1) Grin and bear it; or 2) Grump and lump it. Either way you had to put up with the problem. Now at least there are two nutritional therapies that appear helpful in eliminating the lumps and associated discomfort.

How can you dump a lump? Depending on how much of a coffee-hound or chocoholic you are, therapy can be easy or tough. Lay off the caffeine. Completely. Researchers at the Ohio State University College of Medicine have discovered that the elimination of a group of substances called methylxanthines can get rid of symptoms in many women. Methylxanthines include caffeine, theophylline and theobromine. As you know, coffee and cola drinks are richer in caffeine. Tea is high in theophylline and cocoa is rich in theobromine. Yet all three substances are present in coffee, tea, cola and chocolate as well as in some medications (see 11-1). The easiest way for you to think about it is to eliminate everything that contains caffeine.

The worst part of giving up the stuff is the caffeine-withdrawal headache that may set in soon afterwards. This can nag your noggin for just a day, or for a whole week. I would suggest doing this only when your schedule is favorable to a change involving some discomfort. I also wouldn't wait for the "perfect" week because I truly doubt it exists. Then, while you are "withdrawing," why not pamper yourself in other ways? How about a massage, a pedicure . . . something that's relaxing, to help sooth your sore head?

If you are a purist and absolutely abstain from methylxanthines, your lumps might completely disappear! The pain will probably go away also. But this doesn't happen overnight. It may take up to six months before you are completely symptom-free. Women over 45 years old may have to wait an additional six months before seeing such amazing results. Unfortunately women who smoke may need to wait longer—if any change takes place at all. Nicotine, it turns out, activates substances that support cystic breast disease. So if you want to get rid of the bumps, you'll have to get rid of the butts, too. If you give up along the way and grab a puff or some caffeine perks, your symptoms are likely to return. Keeping the lumps and pain away means staying away from those things that aggravate symptoms.

In the Ohio State study, a few women who were methylxanthine-free were still troubled with symptoms. These women were not smokers, but they were all very athletic and below their ideal body weights. Why such extreme leanness interferes with this particular therapy is now being studied.

Methylxanthines do not cause cystic breast disease. However, their elimination can reduce or completely relieve symptoms. This approach to relief is still not accepted by all physicians. Some doctors may even discourage your trying it out. Since we are only talking about giving up something you don't need anyway (i.e., caffeine, etc.), you may want to give it a whirl. Incidentally, the results of the Ohio State study have subsequently been confirmed and reported in the *Journal of Reproductive Medicine.* This report also noted a diminishment/disappearance of lumps and pain. In addition, less thermal activity was picked up on the mammogram. (In general, there is more thermal activity with a tumorous mass than there is in normal tissue.) Like every other therapy in the books, it works for some, but not all.

Whether or not you junk your java (etc.), you may want to consider a vitamin E supplement. This vitamin can relieve symptoms and normalize abnormal hormone patterns observed in women with fibrocystic breasts. Studies have shown that treatment with a daily dose of 600 IU brought about a relief of symptoms. This included symptoms observed by the patients, and also the more "objective" symptoms that could be measured by their physicians. Six hundred IU's of

Table 11-1: Caffeine Content of Foods and Drugs

ITEM	SERVING SIZE	mg CAFFEINE / SERVING
Beverages:		
Cocoa and Hot Chocolate	8 oz	15
Coffee		
Brewed	5 oz	85-200
Percolated	5 oz	95-125
Dripolated	5 oz	135-150
Instant	5 oz	60
Instant, decaffeinated	5 oz	3
Specialty Coffees		
Cafe Français	1 tsp powder	30
Cafe Vienna	1 tsp powder	30
Orange Cappuccino	1 tsp powder	35
Suisse Mocha	1 tsp powder	30
Tea (5 minute brew)		
Black tea	5 oz	45
Green	5 oz	30
Instant	5 oz	30
Soft Drinks		
Diet Rite	12 oz	36
RC Cola	12 oz	36
Pepsi Light	12 oz	36
Diet Pepsi	12 oz	36
Pepsi-Cola	12 oz	38
Dr. Pepper	12 oz	40
Mr. Pibb	12 oz	40
Sunkist Orange	12 oz	40
Shasta Diet Cola	12 oz	44
Shasta Cola	12 oz	44
Shasta Cherry Cola	12 oz	44
Coca-Cola	12 oz	45
Tab	12 oz	46
Mountain Dew	12 oz	54
Sugar-Free Mr. Pibb	12 oz	60
Nonprescription Drugs		
Anacin	1 tablet	32
Aspirin Compound	1 tablet	32
Bromo-Seltzer	1 tablet	32
Cope	1 tablet	32
Easy-Mens	1 tablet	32
Empirin Compound	1 tablet	32
Exedrin	1 tablet	60
Midol	1 tablet	32
No Doz	1 tablet	100
Pre-Mens	1 tablet	66
Vanquish	1 tablet	42
Many cold preparations	1 tablet	30
Many stimulants	1 tablet	100

Table 11-1 Continued (caffeine content)

ITEM	SERVING SIZE	mg CAFFEINE / SERVING
Prescription Drugs		
APC	1 tablet	32
Cafergot	1 tablet	100
Darvon	1 tablet	40
Fiorinal	1 tablet	40
Migral	1 tablet	50

Based on:

Bunker, M. L.; McWilliams, M. "Caffeine Content of Common Beverages. *J. Am Diet Assocc.*, 1979, 74, 28-31.

Stephenson, P. E. "Physiologic and Psychotropic Effects of Caffeine on Man." *Journal of American Dietetic Association.,* 1977, 71, 248-247.

Anon. "Caffeine Content of Soft Drinks." *Environmental Nutrition Newsletter*, 1983, 6, S-3.

Pennington, J. A.; Church, H. N. *Bowes and Church's Food Values of Portions Commonly Used.* Philadelphia: J. B. Lippincott Company, 1980.

vitamin E is a pretty hefty dose (the RDA is a mere 15 IU) and there is no way you can pick all that up without using a supplement. Even though vitamin E is a fat-soluble vitamin and potentially harmful in large amounts, the dosage used in this study did not produce any apparent adverse effects. Will a lower dose work as well? The answer may make the news soon—researchers are now testing the effectiveness of 150 IU/day.

Vitamin E, say the researchers, is an excellent mode of treatment for cystic breasts. If it turns out that fibrocystic breast disease is truly a precancerous condition, then the chances of cystic breasts advancing to breast cancer may actually be diminished by vitamin E supplementation. It's certainly an exciting prospect, but it's not proven yet.

At this point, you have two strategies for banishing benign breast bumps and pain. There is certainly no harm in giving up caffeine, and to date the suggested vitamin E therapy appears very safe. Not being symptomatic looks like a better option than "lumping and grumping it." You cannot be assured that it will work for you, nor is there any guarantee that it can reduce your higher-than-average breast cancer risk. Adopting either program now is essentially like researching along with the researchers. Who knows what will result as you keep abreast with research in this area? Maybe you'll be able to keep a breast or two healthy!

Make sure you read the next chapter. This is especially important if you have fibrocystic breast disease and/or a history of breast cancer in your family. With a higher likelihood of breast cancer than the average women, you'll find some more suggestions for reducing your risk.

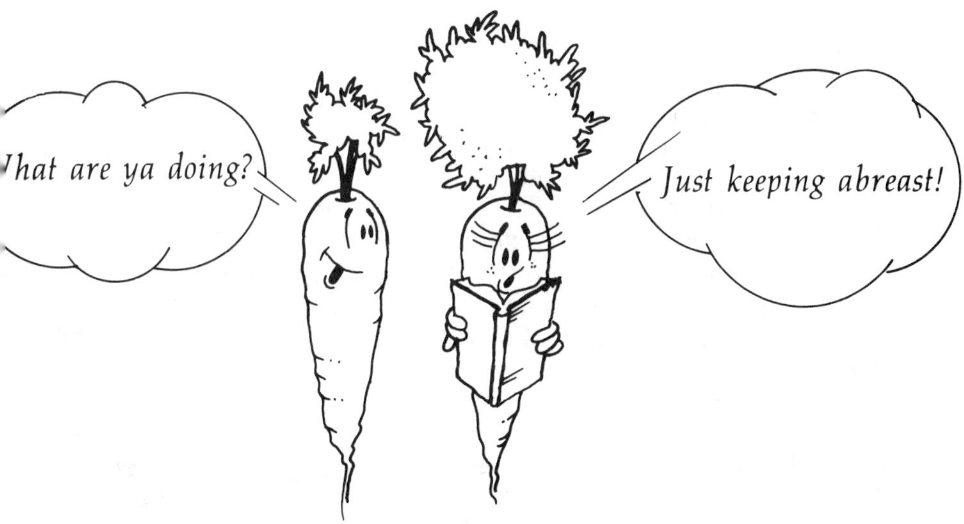

12

BAD BREAST BUMPS

Breast cancer zaps women like crazy. Every year in the USA 100,000 women find out they have it; 30,000 women die because of it. Making the message come a little closer to home is the fact that one out of every 15 women will have breast cancer during her lifetime. So if you don't have it, chances are that someone you know probably will. This is not exactly good news.

Check your breasts out regularly. Look for lumps, nipple changes (discharge, bleeding, inverted nipple), swelling, puckering, dimpling or any distortion in the normal shape of your breast. Do you have any pain, or a skin irritation that persists? If you notice any one of these symptoms, have them examined by a physician.

Who's likely to develop breast cancer? The majority of clues to date suggest that women with "deviations" in the flow and balance of hormones are most susceptible. Overexposure to estrogen seems to be one of the contributing factors. So are alterations in the relationships between hormones during different phases of the lifecycle. In looking at conditions that predispose to breast cancer, you'll be surprised. It turns out that a lot of women are "deviates" (hormonally speaking, that is).

Women who never have children have a higher risk than those who do. In the medical journals, it is noted that women who never marry have a 50% greater chance of getting breast cancer. This higher risk is probably due to the fact that formerly it had been uncommon for single women to bear children and married women not to. As lifestyles change and married women opt for careers instead of kids, and single women choose to have children, the real risk (never married vs. never borne a child) will become apparent. Does sexual activity have an impact? Women who have had none—nuns, for example—have a very high mortality rate for breast cancer. But then again, they've never married nor had children. Women who bear their first full-term child before the age of 18 have about one-third the risk of women whose first full-term delivery does not occur until 35 or later.

Another possible factor in the development of breast cancer which may be closely related to later childbirths is anovulatory cycles—that is, cycles when eggs are *not* shipped out from the ovaries. During these cycles there is a persistent exposure to estrogen without adequate progesterone, and it is that added "abnormal" estrogen exposure that may be the culprit. Long exposure to estrogen would also occur with women who begin menstruating at an early age and go through menopause at a late age. Several other conditions appear to be more common among breast cancer patients, including tenderness and distention of the breast before menstruation, irregular menstrual cycles, a personal history of fibrocystic breast disease and a close relative who has had breast cancer. In the United States, Seventh Day Adventist women (who follow a vegetarian diet) have a lower risk than women chowing down on typical American fare. Women from Westernized cultures run a much higher risk than women in Africa and Asia. As an American, your risk is very high.

Yet if you were Japanese, your risk would be tiny compared to what it is now—provided you still lived in Japan and ate the traditional diet. As chopsticks give way to knives and forks and hamburgers replace sushi, breast cancer incidence begins to climb. And the Westernization of the diet is to blame. This phenomenon is clear when Japanese women migrate east to Hawaii and then to the continental U.S. As they become acculturated and eat typical American foods, their breast cancer risk becomes Americanized as well. Believe it or not, this is good news! How so? Before I tell you, let your fingers do the talking. Look at Figure 12-1.

Put your index finger on the Japanese dot and your right finger on the dot by the USA. Read the caption to the left of the chart, "Age-adjusted breast cancer death rate." Let your fingers slide to the line below each of the dots. Read the caption below the bottom horizontal line."Estimated dietary fat intake (gm/day)."

What are your fingers telling you? The Japanese eat a low-fat diet and have a low risk of breast cancer mortality. Americans, on the other hand, eat a lot more fat and have a much higher breast cancer risk. This is good news, because it says that your breast cancer risk can possibly be altered by varying the amount of fat in your diet. (Although your left finger lucked out this time by pointing to the low-risk groups, your left side is usually less fortunate. For some odd reason, breast cancers occur more frequently in the left breast—even in males when they get mammary cancer (which they rarely do!) Studies on laboratory animals and also of humans indicate that dietary fat plays a major role in breast cancer. Apparently a high-fat intake can alter hormonal metabolism, creating a hormonal environment that is more susceptible to cancer.

In studying the effect of fat, researchers have taken mice and injected them with a carcinogen. One group of mice was then fed low-fat chow and the other, high-fat chow. Then the scientists waited, and watched what happened. Sure enough, the ones with the fatty chow developed lots more mammary tumors. In the meantime, the researchers noticed an alteration in the relationship between estrogen and prolactin, namely that the high-fat diet caused an unusual surge in prolactin, which upset the normal balance between the two. So much for mice, mammaries and hormones. What goes on in people? Similar things!

Figure 12-1. Correlation between age-adjusted death rates from female breast cancer and per capita consumption fat.

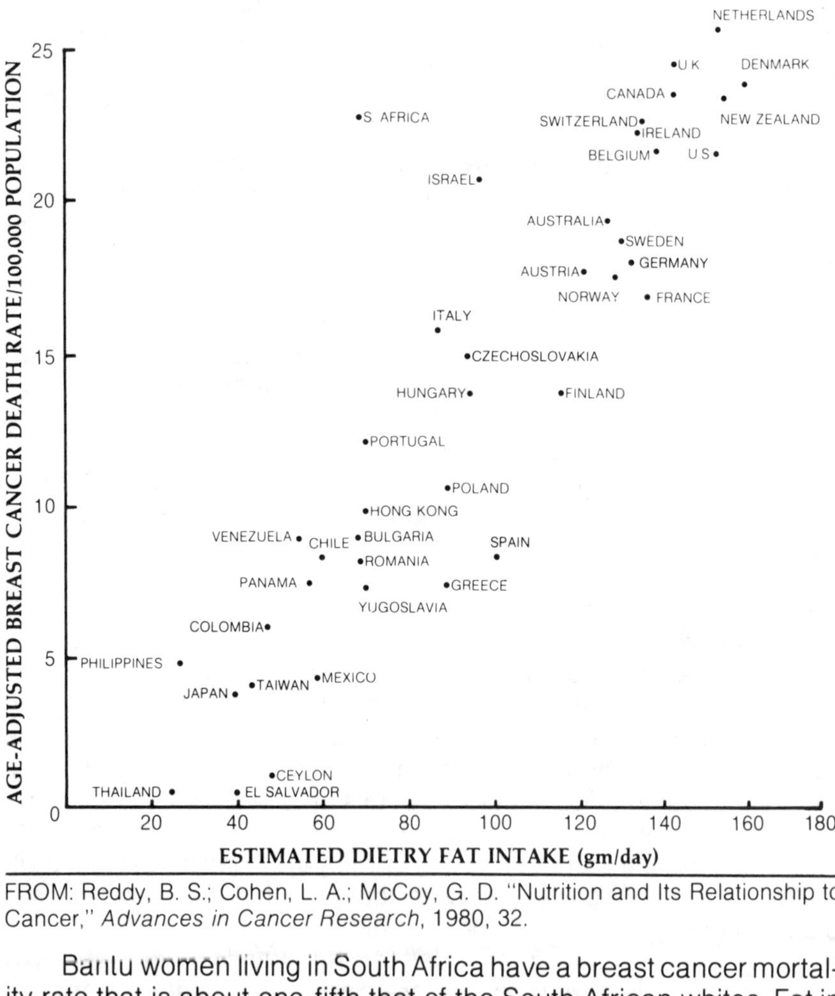

FROM: Reddy, B. S.; Cohen, L. A.; McCoy, G. D. "Nutrition and Its Relationship to Cancer," *Advances in Cancer Research*, 1980, 32.

Bantu women living in South Africa have a breast cancer mortality rate that is about one-fifth that of the South African whites. Fat in the average Bantu diet contributes only 15% of the calories, compared to 40% of the whites' diet. The hormone patterns of the two groups of women are quite different, with the whites having a significantly higher amount of prolactin. Sounds like the mice, doesn't it? Rats! Guess what? The average American woman also gets 40% of her calories as fat, too. No wonder why we run such a high risk of breast cancer!

Even within the USA, there are big differences in eating habits and hormonal patterns. Seventh Day Adventist women (who, as we said, happen to consume a low-fat vegetarian diet) do not have the disparity between estrogen and prolactin to the degree that the rest of the meat-eating population has. What happens if you vary the fat content of an individual's diet? Hormonal patterns change! This means that you may have some control over your breast cancer risk. The high-fat or the low-fat route: Which do you want to take? If you are interested in cutting down the amount of fat you eat, see "Strip and Undress," Chapter 20.

That the balance between estrogen and prolactin strongly influences breast cancer risk becomes even clearer after menopause. Postmenopausal women are at a much higher risk of breast cancer. Now, consider this: With menopause estrogen decreases, thus increasing the already-unbalanced estrogen-prolactin ratio.

It would appear that the greater the disparity, the higher the risk. This helps explain why the postmenopausal American woman's risk is significantly higher than that of her Japanese counterpart. In postmenopausal women who have had breast cancer, recurrence rates are much lower among the Japanese. Their low-fat diet apparently provides some protection. If you have already had this kind of problem, you should consider dropping your fat intake to 20% of your calories. Although the effect of dietary fat restriction on the recurrence rate of breast cancer patients has not been studied and confirmed, several researchers strongly suggest cutting fat intake to levels similar to those of the Japanese and Bantu women.

Diet seems to affect hormonal balance in several ways. A surplus of calories which deposits an excess of personal Crisco (fat in your can) also increases breast cancer risk. Adipose tissue can generate hormones resulting in a disturbance of the natural balance of these regulatory substances. Then again, obesity tends to bring on early menarche (first menstrual period), late menopause, and anovulatory cycles as well—all situations associated with high breast cancer risk. You can see that obesity places a postmenopausal woman in double jeopardy. All this makes flab drab and provides a rather compelling reason to dispose of some adipose. For some sane guidelines on how to lose weight safely, see "Take It Off," Chapter 21.

Fiber is another nutritional component that interacts with hormones. You are probably well aware that fiber provides a natural defense against hemorrhoids and constipation. Its relationship to hormonal status has a lot to do with its action in "Number Two." The relationship is direct: More fiber means bigger stools, and bigger stools carry more estrogen out of the body. That leaves less estrogen available for circulation through the intestine and liver. A dramatic example of dietary-derived differences in estrogen excretion was observed in a study of American women. One group was vegetarian and ate approximately 28 grams of fiber a day. The other group ate more typical fare which provided only 12 grams of fiber. The vegetarian women excreted more than twice as much estrogen via "Number Two."

American Seventh Day Adventists have a breast cancer incidence rate 60-80% that of the rest of the population. Interestingly, women in the lowest-risk populations (where risk is 20-25% that of the USA) eat as much as 40 grams of fiber a day. The high-fiber diet seems to play a protective role. But notice! I said "high-fiber diet," not "fiber.' That's because the observed effect in hormone metabolism might be related to other aspects of the diet as well. In the study where vegetarian women ate 28 grams of fiber, they also ate 25% less fat, a lot less animal protein and less cholesterol. The researchers believe the protection is in the low fat/high fiber combo! How are your F-ing habits? (See "Strip and Undress," Chapter 20, and "Fiber for Fluffies," Chapter 19, to find out!)

In addition to the fat-fiber-hormone routine, another nutrient also helps guard against breast cancer: selenium. Available evidence suggests that a lack of dietary selenium increases cancer susceptibility. Where ambient selenium levels are low, cancer rates run high. The Japanese seem to win here, too. Their average daily selenium intake is about 300 mcg, just about double the typical American consumption. In addition to these epidemiological observations, studies on laboratory animals also indicate that selenium plays a protective role against breast cancer. A strain of mice which is genetically inbred to spontaneously develop this kind of malignancy have an 80-100% mortality rate from the disease. However, researchers have shown that supplementing their drinking water with selenium reduces their mortality rate to about 10%!

You can find selenium in seafood, organ meats (especially kidney), very lean meat, poultry, whole-grain breads and cereals, garlic, mushrooms, asparagus and in yeast grown on selenium-rich soil. Most plants don't need selenium and so they are not reliable sources. Also, the selenium content of soil varies, so that animals that graze on selenium-poor soil will have a low content. So will plants that are grown there. This means that vegetarians may not pick up an adequate amount from their diet. In view of this, a supplement of 50-100 mcg/day has been recommended. There is no specific Recommended Dietary Allowance for selenium, although an intake of 50-200 mcg/day is considered "safe and adequate." Judging from, available data, it appears that a higher intake (200 mcg) is a better bet.

Table 12-1: Selenium Content of Food

FOOD	SERVING SIZE	mg SELENIUM / SERVING
Protein Foods:		
Beef (round steak)	1 oz.	9.5
Beef, ground, raw	1 oz	5.5
Beef liver, raw	1 oz	12.0
Beef kidney, raw	1 oz	43.0
Pork (chop, raw)	1 oz	6.5
Pork kidney, raw	1 oz	53.0
Lamb (chop, raw)	1 oz	5.0
Lamb kidney	1 oz	40.0
Average meat (excluding kidney & liver)	1 oz	6.5
Chicken (breast)	1 oz	3.0
Chicken (leg)	1 oz	4.0
Average Chicken	1 oz	3.5
Lobster tail	1 oz	18.5
Shrimp, shelled, deveined	1 oz	16.5
Cod fillet	1 oz	12.0
Flounder fillet	1 oz	9.5
Oysters	1 oz	18.0
Average fish (excluding shellfish	1 oz	11.0
Egg	1 large	6.0
Cheese, American	1 oz	2.5
Cheese, cottage	4 oz (½ cup)	6.0
Cheese, Swiss	1 oz	3.0
Average hard cheese	1 oz	3.0
Grains:		
Bread, white	1 slice	6.0
Bread, whole-wheat	1 slice	15.5
Cereal, barley, dry	½ cup	12.0
Cereal (Cheerios)	1 cup	11.0
Cereal (corn flakes)	1 cup	.5
Cereal (oats, quick-cooked)	¾ cup	3.0
Cereal, rice puffed	1 cup	.5
Cereal (wheatena, cooked)	2/3 cup	7.0
Cereal (Wheaties)	1 cup	3.0
Flour, white	¼ cup	5.0
Flour, whole-wheat	¼ cup	19.0
Noodles, egg, dry	½ cup	20.0
Rice, polished, cooked	¾ cup	9.0
Rice, brown, cooked	¾ cup	11.0
Vegetables:		
Carrots, fresh	1 large	2.0
Garlic, fresh	1 clove	.5
Mushrooms, fresh	4 large	13.0
Radishes, fresh	5 small	2.0

Derived from V. C. Morris and O. A. Levander, "Selenium Content of Foods," *Journal of Nutrition*, 100: 1383-1388, 1970.

Check out Table 12-1 to see how your selenium intake adds up. If it's low, figure out what foods you can add to increase it. In addition, you may benefit from a supplement. Make sure the source is from "yeast grown on selenium-rich soil". Check the label for the symbol of a pill, which notes "certified natural high-selenium yeast." L-selenomethionine is also a good source. Other forms of selenium (i.e., selenium salts) are not readily used by your body, and may be less effective. One thing you need to remember is that high doses of selenium are toxic. Even though it is protective in relatively small doses, huge doses are counterproductive.

Now you have four steps you can take to lessen your risk of breast cancer. First of all, cut down on fats. Keep your fat calories between 20-30% of your total calorie intake. Then, eat plenty of fiber-containing foods. Lose weight if you are too heavy and make sure your diet is rich in selenium.

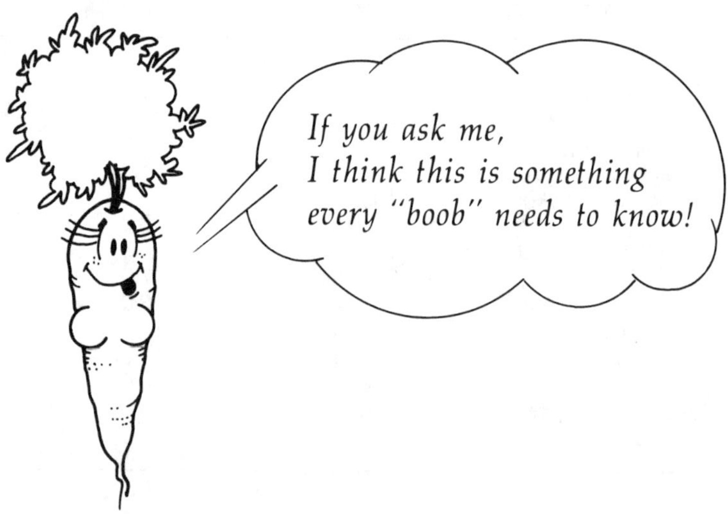
If you ask me,
I think this is something
every "boob" needs to know!

13

FEMALE FLASHERS

Sometime between the ages of 40 and 50 a lot of women become "flashers"—as they go through menopause, they may get hot flashes and experience a variety of other symptoms, including depression, fatigue and insomnia. This may or may not happen to you.

Not all women are troubled by the classical menopausal symptoms. For those who are, estrogen therapy is often prescribed. However, this form of therapy is not appropriate for women with a personal history of cancer, because estrogen might activate dormant cancer cells. Many menopausal women would prefer not to take estrogens, yet want relief from the hot flashes and the rest.

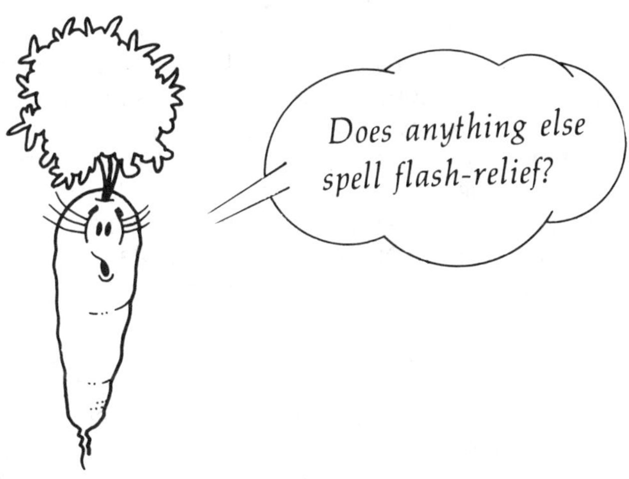

Perhaps Vitamin E may do the trick.

During the mid-1940s and early 1950s, vitamin E was studied as a potential substitute for estrogen therapy in patients with previous history of cancer. In one of the first studies, relatively low daily doses (about 10-30 IU, with the dose depending on the severity of symptoms) were administered to a group of women with menopausal symptoms. Some were going through natural menopause, while others had "artificial" menopause resulting from surgical removal of the ovaries, and/or radium therapy. All of the women responded well! Hot flashes and drenching perspiration were either greatly improved or else completely disappeared. Moreover, almost all the women experienced a positive change in mood and outlook.

The exciting aspect of this alternative therapy was its lack of side effects when compared with estrogen treatment. Hormone therapy can produce a variety of undesirable reactions, including headache, nausea, vomiting, dizziness, soreness of the breasts, pelvic pain and vaginal bleeding. The real plus was that vitamin E was as effective as estrogen in relieving the menopausal symptoms . . . without increasing cancer risk!

Subsequent studies also showed similar results. The researchers concluded that vitamin E was "undoubtedly effective" in treating hot flashes and some of the associated symptoms, and was considered a valuable remedy for women for whom estrogen therapy is not advised. In spite of this success, use of vitamin E is sometimes frowned upon by practitioners — they are afraid that large doses of it can be harmful. Yet a recent review indicates that daily intakes up to 600 IU are innocuous in most people. Dosage levels used during the vitamin E/menopause trials were as low as 10 IU and, for the most part, not higher than 100 IU, well within the accepted range of safety.

In 1958 a physician writing into the Q&A section of the *Journal of the American Medical Association* asked what medication was suitable for a 42-year-old woman who was experiencing menopausal symptoms brought on by surgery for cancer. This was the answer he got: "The use of alpha-tocopherol (vitamin E), 25 mg. given three times a day, is recommended. Estrogens are definitely contraindicated in individuals who have been treated for carcinoma, due to the fact that they may activate dormant cells to malignant phases. Alpha-tocopherol causes no such stimulation of dormant cells which may have this propensity. This consultant has had some success with this medication; it is recommended with the belief that it has definite value in diminishing or causing absence of hot flashes." (*JAMA,* 1958, 167, p. 1806.)

"Since the 1950's, vitamin E therapy for menopausal symptoms has dropped out of vogue. In the meantime, a safe form of estrogen replacement therapy has become fairly common practice. Yet some women, in seeking relief from hot flashes, would rather not take hormones. While research done 30-40 years ago indicates vitamin E's effectiveness in some women, new studies need to be done to clarify the benefits of vitamin therapy. Women who want to try vitamin E should keep their dose within safe limits, i.e. 25-600 IU of d-alpha tocopherol daily. If you are interested in menopause and mid-life wellness, see the resource section for more information on the Center for Climacteric Studies.

14

BREAKING UP

Contrary to an oldie goldie, breaking up is *not* hard to do. It's easy and it happens all the time. Broken bones, fractures, and spinal deformities, such as Dowager's Hump, are all associated with osteoporosis.

Osteoporosis is a condition characterized by a demineralization of the bones. The steady loss of calcium from the bones over a long period of time causes bones to become brittle. In advanced stages, osteoporosis is marked by back pain and a decrease in body height. When calcium loss is severe enough to weaken vertebrae, the spine may crush from simple exertion or just from the weight of the body. It's the crushing of the vertebrae that leads to deformities such as dowager's hump. Osteoporosis is usually the underlying cause for the 190,000 broken hips among the elderly each year. It's also responsible for 70% of the 1,000,000 bone fractures that occur yearly. Just about everyone knows of someone's Aunt Nellie who fell and either fractured or broke a hip.

You stop growing up when you're about 18 years old, but your bones continue to grow in density until you're 35. Throughout your life there is a constant turnover of calcium in your bones. Some is deposited each day; some is lost. When losses consistently exceed the amount laid down, your bones gradually become thinner.

Ninety-nine percent of the calcium in your body is in the bone. The other one percent maintains the health and function of the nerves and muscles. When calcium intake is inadequate, bone calcium is sacrificed to support the work of the other one percent.

When your diet replenishes lost calcium, your bones remain strong. When it doesn't, a tiny amount of calcium is mobilized out of the bone. Small losses add up. After 20 or 30 years there's a remarkable decrease in bone mass, so much so that one day you might do what old Aunt Nellie did—break a hip!

By the time osteoporosis is discovered, a lot of bone degeneration has already taken place. Current treatments seem to arrest bone loss. Needless to say, the best way to deal with osteoporosis is to prevent it. Several factors influence its development: A diet that favors calcium loss is one. Lack of exercise is another, as is the decrease in estrogen that naturally occurs in post-menopausal women.

Although osteoporosis occurs in men and women, postmenopausal women run the highest risk of developing it. One fourth of women over 60 years of age have some degree of osteoporosis. Although the postmenopausal hormonal changes spur calcium loss, not all women will develop this bone problem. However, for women in this age group, inadequate calcium intakes are quite common. Many older women are sedentary. The combination of decreased estrogen and poor dietary and exercise habits is bad for bones.

Several dietary factors have an impact on the health and strength of your bones. Calcium intake might be adequate (RDA=800 mg) yet an excessive consumption of protein (especially from animal products) speeds up calcium loss. To maintain calcium balance, people eating large amounts of protein require more calcium than those who eat less. In Asia, where protein intakes are adequate (not inordinate), bone strength is maintained on 400-500 mg/day; degenerative bone disease is uncommon. In the U.S., where calcium intake often falls short of the recommended amount and protein intake is at least double the requirements, osteoporosis is very common. A wise preventive measure would be to match your protein intake to your actual requirements (see "The Curse," Chapter 9) and eat a variety of calcium-containing foods daily.

If you like milk products, two servings a day will provide nearly all the calcium you need. The remainder is easy to pick up from other foods. Carefully review the list: see Table 14-1. There are a surprising number of foods that contain hefty amounts of calcium. Although some foods on the list only contain 20-50 mg, a few of them each day does add up!

Several factors other than protein intake affect bone health. Sugar and alcohol cause a sharp, albeit transient, rise in urinary calcium excretion. With 24% of our national daily calories coming from sugar, it's likely that the sweets are not a treat for our bones. To find out more about your sugar consumption, see "Getting Stoned," Chapter 15. That reminds me: Alcoholism is also believed to play a role in osteoporosis.

There has been some concern that a high-fiber diet interferes with calcium absorption. That's true, to an extent. So don't go hog wild and fill up your trough with bran. By the same token, it's smart to look at the bone health of people who eat a high-fiber diet. Postmenopausal Seventh Day Adventist women who have been eating a well-selected vegetarian diet (typically high in fiber) for over 20 years have healthier bones than omnivorous women in the same age bracket. This kind of study suggests that it's the dietary *pattern* that can make or break your bones, not necessarily one isolated factor.

An adequate supply of vitamin D is also essential for calcium

Table 14-1: Calcium Content of Foods
Recommended Dietary Allowance:
800 mg
1200 mg if pregnant
1200 mg if breastfeeding

FOOD	SERVING SIZE	mg CALCIUM PER SERVING
Breads and Cereals:		
Biscuits	2″ in diameter	40
Bread	1 slice	20
Cornbread	2″ square	55
Muffin	1 average	40
Oatmeal, cooked	1 cup	15
Pancake	4″ in diameter	45
Pancake, buckwheat	4″ in diameter	100
Pasta, cooked	1 cup	15
Tortilla, corn	6″ in diameter	60
Waffle	5½″ in diameter	85
Whole-wheat cereal, cooked	1 cup	20
Dairy Products:		
Cheese, American	1 oz	200
Cheese, cheddar	1 oz	210
Cheese, cottage	½ cup	105
Cheese, mozzarella	1 oz	145
Cheese, ricotta, part-skim	½ cup	337
Cheese, Swiss	1 cup	260
Milk, buttermilk	1 cup	300
Milk, dry instant	¼ cup powder	195
Milk, evaporated	½ cup	250
Milk, skim or lowfat	1 cup	300
Milk, whole	1 cup	290
Milk, goat's	1 cup	315
Ice cream	½ cup	130
Yogurt, lowfat	1 cup	300
Fruits:		
Average piece if not listed	½ cup	10-15
Blackberries	1 cup	45
Figs, dried	5 medium	125
Orange, fresh	3″ in diameter	60
Orange, fresh	3⅝″ in diameter	95
Prunes, dried and cooked	8 medium	60
Prunes, dried, uncooked	8 medium	90
Watermelon	1/16 melon	65
Legumes, Nuts, Seeds, Soy Products:		
Almonds, shelled	¼ cup	25
Garbanzo beans, cooked	3½ oz	75
Peanuts	¼ cup	45
Peanut butter	2 tablespoons	20
Soybeans, cooked	2/3 cup	60
Soybean curd (Tofu)	2½ × 2 × 2¾	300

Table 14-1 Continued (Calcium Content)
Legumes, Nuts, Seeds, Soy Products:

FOOD	SERVING SIZE	mg CALCIUM PER SERVING
Soybean milk	1 cup	55
Soybean nuts	½ oz	35
Sesame seeds, unhulled	2 tablespoons	200
Sunflower seeds	3½ oz	120
Seafood:		
Herring, kippered	3½ oz/1 small fish	65
Mackerel, canned	½ cup	195
Sardines	3½ oz	450
Salmon, canned	½ cup	195
Scallops, steamed	3½ oz	115
Shrimp, fried	3½ oz	70
Vegetables:		
Average vegetable not listed	½ cup	20
Artichoke	1 (edible portion)	50
Beans, green or yellow, cooked	1 cup	55
Broccoli, steamed	1 cup	130
Cabbage, steamed	1 cup	75
Collards, steamed	½ cup	205
Dandelion greens, steamed	½ cup	185
Kale, steamed	¾ cup	180
Lettuce (romaine)	¼ head	70
Mustard greens, steamed	1 cup	275
Okra, cooked	1 cup	90
Parsnips, steamed	1 cup	90
Squash, acorn, baked	½	60
Sweet potato	1 large	50
Turnip greens, steamed	1 cup	275
Miscellaneous:		
Custard	½ cup	130
Molasses, blackstrap	1 tablespoon	115
Pudding	½ cup	145

Adapted from: Pennington, J. A.; Church, H. N. *Bowes and Church's Food Values of Portions Commonly Used.* Philadelphia: J. B. Lippincott Company, 1980.

absorption. The recommended intake is 400 IU, not all of which needs to come from your food. Getting outside in the sunshine is another pleasant way to pick up some vitamin D. Just 20 minutes' exposure of your hands and face gives you your daily requirement. Darker-skinned people need more time for the same effect.

As long as we're talking about getting outside, make sure you go out and do some physical activity each day. People who are immobilized or in weightless environments lose a lot of calcium. So do people who fail to exercise regularly. Doing a few leg lifts in front of your TV is not enough. For exercise to exert a protective effect on your bone mass, it must be weight-bearing. Walking, jogging, tennis are all excellent!

Osteoporosis is not just a problem reserved for older ladies. A leading calcium researcher believes that available evidence indicates that a dietary calcium deficiency can accelerate bone loss in young people (especially women) as young as age 25. Even younger men now seem to be developing osteoporosis. In a recent study, signs of bone deterioration were observed in a group of young men. Their problem? Too much dietary protein! Apparently, urinary calcium losses increased in direct proportion to the amount of protein they consumed. If you're a man and think that huge hunks of meat are macho, you'd better reconsider. Excessive amounts of protein foods, particularly those of animal origin, can deteriorate your bones! (Figure out your actual protein needs; see Table 9-1 in "The Curse," Chapter 9.) Cut down on the size of your meat portions: add a few vegetarian-style entrees each week. The benefits will outweigh what seems to be a slight sacrifice right now. You'll probably lose some weight, and you'll also reduce your risk of heart disease and prostatic cancer as well. What do you think?

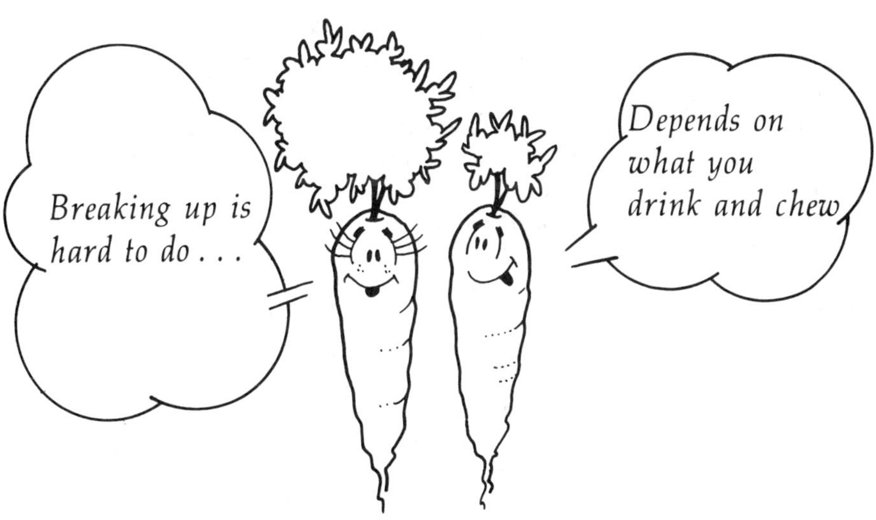
Breaking up is hard to do . . .
Depends on what you drink and chew

15

GETTING STONED

Did you ever have sex when you were stoned? (Kidney stoned, that is!) Not that it's completely impossible, but it has got to be downright uncomfortable. Sometimes you can be getting stoned and not know it. But the odds are you'll eventually feel something.

Typical symptoms include back pain, or suprapubic pain if the stone is in your bladder. The pain can be in your abdominal area or along your ureter. Often the pain hits in your "tender region" and inner thigh. The pain is not constant but tends to come intermittently and very, very sharply. (The textbooks say it's "excruciating pain!") Sometimes there's nausea, vomiting, and a bloated feeling in your belly. Chills, fever, bloody urine and a need to "go" frequently are common, particularly as the stone travels down your ureter.

Although most of us think of them as kidney stones, their real name is urinary calculi. "Stone" for short. One out of every thousand persons goes to the hospital every year because of them. There are quite a few reasons why people get stoned. What you eat and/or drink is among them.

Did you ever wonder why you were supposed to drink those 8-10 glasses of water every day? (Soda pop won't do—read on.) One reason is to keep your urine fairly dilute. When you're dehydrated, the proportion of potential stone constituents to fluid greatly increases, and so does the likelihood of a stone precipitating out of your urine. Here's a rather simplified way of looking at it: Think of a glass of iced tea. It can easily accommodate a teaspoon of sugar. The sugar dissolves and becomes part of the iced tea. OK, now think of the same size glass, only this time you're putting in six teaspoons of sugar. Some of it dissolves, and some of it remains. You have two choices: Let the sugar settle out. Or add more tea till all the sugar dissolves. When your fluid intake is limited, you increase your own chances of getting stoned.

Vitamin deficiency, specifically an inadequate amount of vitamin B-6, is another fairly common cause of stones. Vitamin B-6 deficiency is not that uncommon either. For that matter, our "typical" dietary pattern favors it. An excessive amount of sugar, white flour products and fats can eventually bring on a B-6 deficiency. Superimpose this on a high protein intake and B-6 problems are even more likely.

Believe it or not, the American diet looks like this: 42% fat; 24% sugar. Over one-half the starches that we eat are refined. Besides that, most people are eating double or triple the amount of protein they need. Recently there's been a big push to include more whole grains, fruits and veggies. That's a huge improvement over the high protein fad several years back. Remember? Protein was a buzzword for selling anything from dog food to shampoo. (I often thought automobile manufacturers should have introduced a high-protein line of cars to boost sales.) Is your protein intake reasonable or ridiculously high? (See Table 9-1 in "The Curse," Chapter 9, and figure it out for yourself.)

As mentioned in "The Pill," Chapter 8, the best sources of B-6 include: lean meat, liver, dark-green leafy vegetables, potatoes and sweet potatoes, egg yolk, fish and shellfish, legumes (dried peas and beans, kidney beans, lentils, etc.), peanuts and peanut butter, prunes, raisins and whole-grain breads and cereals. A lot of B-6 is lost during the refining of grains as well as in the canning and freezing of vegetables, and in the canning of meat and fish.

Oh, just for the record: If you think a huge steak will satisfy your B-6 requirement, think again. Over 70% of the calories in a steak are fat, and a 12-oz. steak contains 84 grams of protein, substantially more than you need all day! There's no need to get rid of the meat completely. However, smaller portions of leaner cuts is a smart idea.

Calcium and oxalate are substances normally found in the urine. Under certain circumstances, however, the calcium and oxalate combine to form relatively insoluble crystals. The crystals, calcium oxalate stones, are not necessarily caused by too much calcium. Apparently, inadequate B-6 spurs their formation. In a recent study, stone patients were given 10 mg of B-6 for 180 days. A significant decrease in calcium and oxalate was noted. For the first 90 days, the patients were marginally deficient in B-6. However, the deficiency was eventually cleared up by the vitamin supplementation. Vitamin-replacement therapy is effective. But why create the deficiency in the first place? By eating well, you can avert stones that occur because of an inadequate B-6 supply.

Another nutrient helpful in preventing stone formation is magnesium. Supplementation with 200 mg of it a day seemed to do the trick for some patients. The RDA is 350-400 mg/day for adults. Not too surprisingly, a lot of us aren't getting enough. In fact, dietary surveys show that self-selected diets often contain as little as 200-250 mg/day. Why? Because it's not found in sugar and fats (66% of the typical American diet is from sugar and fat!) Besides there are large

Table 15-1: Sugar Content of Foods

How much sweet stuff do you usually eat? If your eating habits are fairly consistent day to day, a one-day review might give you a reasonable idea. However, it's probably best to keep track of your sweet tooth for a week.

The sugar content of the foods listed below is given in tablespoons. The average American eats twelve of them a day! Do you?

FOOD	SERVING SIZE	SUGAR CONTENT TABLESPOONS	TABLESPOONS I ATE
Cake, iced	1 piece	4	
Candy bar	1 average	1	
Cereal, presweetened	½ cup	1	
Cookies	2 small	1	
Doughnut, glazed	1	2	
Doughnut, plain	1	1	
Fruit, canned	½ cup	1	
Fruit "drink"	8 oz	2	
Fudge	1¼" cube	2	
Ice cream	½ cup	1	
Ice cream cone (the cone)	1	1	
Ice cream sundae	1	4	
Jello	1 cup	3	
Jelly, marmelade or jam	1 tablespoon	1	
Lemonade	1 cup	2	
Milk, chocolate	8 oz	1	
Pie, custard cream	1 slice	2	
Pie, fruit	1 slice	3	
Popsicle	twin bar	2	
Pudding	½ cup	1	
Roll, sweet	1 small	1	
Sherbert	½ cup	2	
Soda	12 oz	3	
Sugar	1 tablespoon	1	
Syrup	1 tablespoon	1	
Yogurt, flavored	8 oz	2	
		MY TOTAL FOR TODAY =	______

losses of magnesium from wheat when it's processed into white flour. There's none in sugar. There's none in fat. Nor is there any in alcohol. When eaten excessively, refined foods can cause a "relative" deficiency; need surpasses supply.

Magnesium is found in most of the foods that are rich in B-6: whole grains, nuts, legumes, peanuts and peanut butter and green leafy vegetables. In addition to lessening the possibility of kidney stones, magnesium works to prevent broken hearts. Altered heart rhythms, heart attack and something called sudden death ischemic heart disease are caused, in part, by an inadequate magnesium supply. So eat your greens and beans. (If you're worried about the explosive potential of the latter, look at it this way: Give a fart for your heart!)

Is it any surprise that some researchers have given both magnesium and B-6 to frequent stone formers? In one study, this combo cut calculi occurrence well over 80%! In 1978 British researchers found that diets high in refined carbohydrates (sugar, white flour) tend to encourage stone formation. That does not seem too surprising, considering the impact of refining on the B-6 and magnesium content of foods. This is just one of the troubles with "empty calorie" foods and by the way, the term "empty calories" doesn't mean "without calories."

Calories provide energy, something we all need. However, when your body transforms food energy into energy you can use, it needs the presence of vitamins and minerals. They serve as catalysts, enabling the proper reactions to occur and the proper byproducts to be formed. When there's an inordinate amount of calories and an insufficient supply of vitamins and minerals, things don't work correctly. Biochemical reactions are not completed properly, abnormal byproducts are produced and your wellbeing is jeopardized. (Incidentally, B-6 and magnesium both play central roles in energy metabolism.)

Do you have any idea how much sugar you're eating? Look at Table 15-1 to find out. Soda pop is, unquestionably, the most popular single supplier of sugar. So while drinking a lot of fluids is helpful in reducing stone formation, it's not smart to "pop" a stone. If you do, you might have to drop a stone!

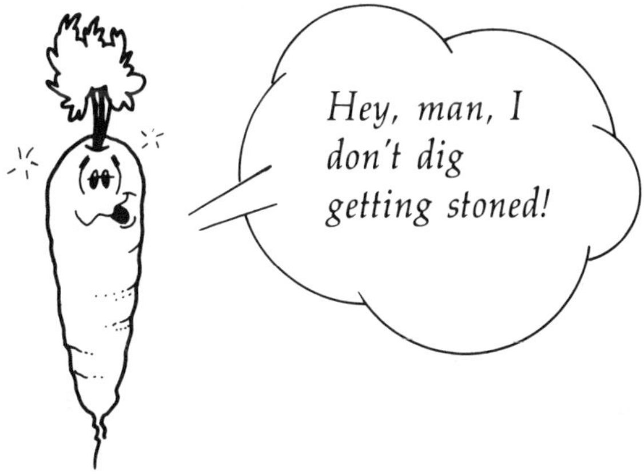

16

HERPES

Herpes is in the news a lot these days. But it's nothing new: Even the Romans and Greeks had it. In fact, the word "herpes" comes from the Greek meaning "to creep." However if this creepy virus were to be named today, it would more appropriately have to come from a word meaning "to spread like wildfire!" Herpes is not creeping any more; it's dashing from person to person at the alarming rate of 500,000 people per year. Supposedly over five million people in the U.S. have the problem. That makes it a popular STD. (STD means "sexually transmitted disease." In case you haven't heard, "STD" is "in"; "VD" is "out.")

Although there are over five types of herpes viruses, the contemporary headliner is Herpes Simplex II—the kind that is often, but not always, transmitted by sexual contact. (Herpes virus can apparently survive up to four hours on an inanimate object, although no one knows for sure if this is true of the Simplex Type II variety. So heed Mom's old warning about public toilet seats!)

Once you come in contact with the virus, it takes about six days for the blisters to appear. Just before they make their appearance, you'll feel a burning, itchy sensation on the infected area. Then the lesion shows up, and it is not very attractive. It's painful, emotionally and physically. Herpes is only infective when it is in the active stage. (It's so spreadable, it's incredible.) But the miserable thing about herpes is that it doesn't go away. Instead, it hides out in nerve cells and reappears when the body's defenses are down. Emotional stress can trigger a recurrence. (Just imagine what happens when you get really upset about having herpes. . . .) So can other factors such as smoking, sunburn, wind, trauma, fever and even menstruation.

Herpes can cause some other trouble, including eye infections, encephalitis and pneumonia. The worst complication of female genital herpes is infection of the newborn during delivery: The virus can spread rapidly throughout the baby's system. More than half of the estimated 1,000 children born with herpes each year will die, and the rest will be permanently brain-damaged! Caesarian sections should be performed on women who have had a herpes outbreak within two weeks of delivery. The presence of herpes also seems to greatly increase the risk of cervical cancer. So if you have the virus, make sure you check in with your physician for a Pap smear twice a year. Keep your cervix well nourished. (See "High-Class Pap," Chapter 3.)

One of the biggest problems with herpes is finding a cure. There is none . . . yet! You may have heard that L-Lysine, an amino acid supplement, is helpful. A few articles have appeared in the medical journals suggesting that lysine is effective in the treatment of herpes. However, other studies give conflicting reports. No matter what you have heard, one thing is certain: it doesn't cure the stuff. So far, nothing seems to knock out the virus that's lodged in the nerve cells.

In 1978 a clinical trial was carried out on people who claimed to be suffering from herpes. As reported in the medical journal *Dermatologica*, a group of people with recurrent herpes were given 800-1,000 mg of L-lysine hydrochloride daily during a period of overt infection. When the infection subsided, they were given 300-500 mg daily as a maintenance dose. In addition, the patients were asked to avoid foods that are high in amino acid arginine, mainly nuts, seeds, chocolate. (It has been postulated that a high lysine:arginine ratio suppresses herpesvirus growth.) They were followed by the researchers for as little as three months to as long as two years. During that time, none of the patients reported any adverse reaction to the lysine therapy. What did it do for the herpes?

According to the researchers, lysine therapy resulted in the disappearance of pain overnight in virtually every instance; the initial sore stayed put and did not creep to other sites. A few patients who previously had to lose work because of the severity of their symptoms found that the lysine rapidly controlled the virus outbreaks. Continued use of lysine was accompanied by a continued suppression of herpes. There were fewer recurrences. Most patients found that they were symptom-free . . . provided they continued taking lysine. Whenever they stopped taking the medication, the herpes would return within one week to one month. Those who had established a maintenance dose would "break through" whenever they reduced their dose. While the maintenance dose varied from individual to individual, nearly everyone went recurrence-free on 500 mg lysine a day. A stinging pain signalled that herpes was ready to make an "encore." Five hundred to 1000 mg of lysine taken at that time could snuff out a fresh outbreak.

Because patients experienced a relapse when they discontinued the lysine therapy, this amino acid can be considered a herpes-suppressant, not a cure. Some failures with lysine therapy have been attributed to an inadequate dose, or to the use of plain lysine or D-lysine. D-lysine an ineffective form of lysine; plain lysine, a mixture of the "D" and "L" forms, is much less potent than pure L-lysine.

The researchers also suggest that herpes patients avoid foods high in arginine. They observed that those eating a lot of arginine-rich foods needed more L-lysine for herpes control than those who used milk and other lysine-rich foods. (See Table 16-1.)

Table 16-1 Lysine and Arginine Content of Foods

High-Lysine Foods:	
Beef	Fish
Brewer's yeast	Milk (cow, goat, human)
Chicken	Pork
Cheese (all types)	Shellfish
Egg	Soybeans and other beans
High-Arginine Foods:	
Carob	Garbanzo beans (chickpeas)
Cereals (Wheat, oatmeal, rice)	Peanut butter
Chocolate	Nuts (all kinds)
Cocoa	Raisins
Coconut	Seeds
Corn	

It was this particular study that spurred a lot of public interest in lysine. Yet as long as we are discussing this particular research piece, it would be worthwhile to look at why it seemed to produce such successful results. A closer look at the design of the study reveals several major flaws.

For instance, the sores were not cultured to ascertain the existence of herpesvirus. And there was not a second group of subjects who received a placebo. If this study had been performed under ideal research conditions, one group should have received a placebo and the other, lysine. The results would have been more objective.

In 1984, such a well-designed study was reported in the Archives of Dermatology. What did these researchers find out? Believe it or not, they concluded that lysine was NO more effective than the placebo. Although the final word is probably not in on lysine, it appears that it is not as promising as originally suggested.

Suppose you decide to use it. Are there any serious effects? Although very high doses of lysine (10-40 grams/day) can produce abdominal cramps and diarrhea, the suggested "anti-herpes" dose of one gram has not been shown to produce these effects. However, this does not mean it is completely safe. Several studies indicate that a high lysine:arginine ratio in the diet may raise blood cholesterol levels and, subsequently, increase heart disease risk. Whether or not lysine supplements heighten risk of heart disease has yet to be explored. Keep in mind, though, that a life-long dependency on the stuff may hold hidden danger.

If you think herpes is your bed-bug, your best bet would be to see your physician A.S.A.P. While there is no cure, the new drug acyclovir can take the "creeps" out of your problem and prevent it from creeping on to someone else.

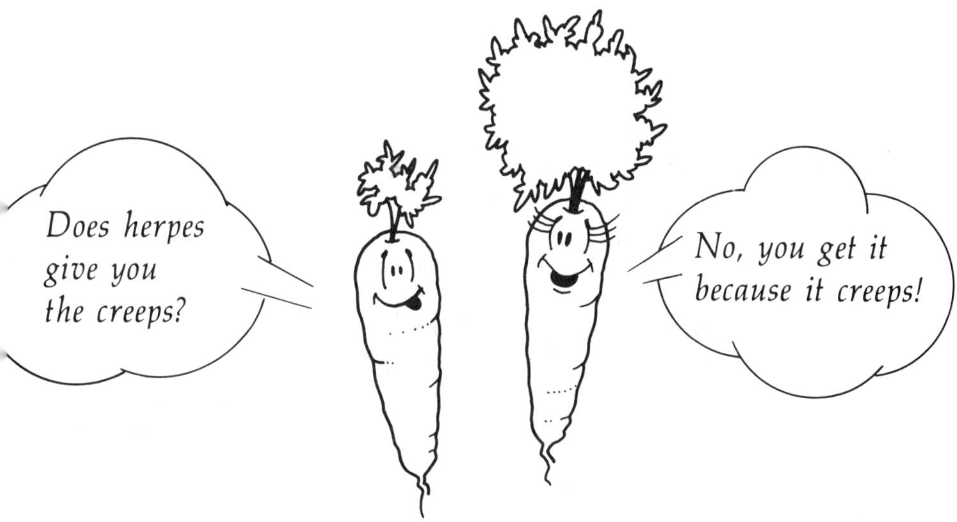
Does herpes give you the creeps?
No, you get it because it creeps!

17

HEADACHES

"Not tonight, honey. I have a headache!" Sound familiar?

Sad words. They dampen the spirit. But pity the one with the pounding head. Chances are he or she has no idea where it came from, unless it's the common hangover variety. Yet not all headaches are a throbbing reminder of a few too many. Some everyday foods can spur head pain.

Admittedly, when it comes to noggin naggers, alcoholic beverages head the list. Alcohol is a vasodilator and expands the arteries coming into your head, allowing more blood to come rolling on through. That onrush of blood can trigger a headache. But that's not the only reason why booze bangs brains. Other properties of spirited beverages, "tailings" and "fusel oil," are powerful migraine producers. You may never have heard of either of these, but you probably like them because they impart the characteristic flavor you enjoy.

If your head aches from alcohol, then vodka might be best for you. It's pure ethyl alcohol and has none of the migraine-producing amines found in the tailings and fusel oil of other liquors. The worst thing to drink is red wine. Full of histamine, it can really start your head pounding. Red wine, brandy and liquers all hit your head pretty hard, followed by (from worst to best) gin to light scotch.

Caffeine causes headaches in some, relieves headaches in others. Caffeine is a vasoconstrictor, so it's useful in heading off any headache associated with vasodilation. During the first stage of a migraine, caffeine might counter the attack. But timing is of the essence: if taken too late the caffeine will not be able to curtail the pain. The potential hangover sufferer might like to know that coffee and three aspirins before bedtime may curb tomorrow's "*caput throbiensis.*" Now really! Why not prevent it a little earlier than that by drinking more moderately in the first place?

Too much caffeine can get your head throbbing, too. But don't reach for a caffeine-containing analgesic (Anacin, aspirin compound, Empirin Compound, Excedrin) which may temporarily quiet the pain. Unfortunately it can also lead to a vicious cycle of recurring headaches. Now if you decide to give up the stuff altogether, you'll suffer head pain for a day—or a week, depending on how much of a java hound you are. Caffeine is, after all, a stimulant. So don't expect to withdraw from it without some withdrawal symptoms. Some people have a mild withdrawal crisis each weekend. During the week, they gulp down coffee as fast as the office urn produces it. When the weekend comes they may only have one or two cups a day, quite a change from their usual ten or twenty. A headache sets in. It might be mistaken for problems with weekend home life rather than for a caffeine mini-withdrawal.

If you're a chocolate lover, you won't like this news: Chocolate contains a powerful vasoactive substance, phenythlyamine, which can produce headaches in susceptible people within a half hour! Take heart; not everyone has a sensitivity to it. See Table 11-1 for the caffeine content of foods and drugs.

Other favorites may also hurt your head. Take cheese. The aged varieties, in particular, contain tyramine. So if you pack some cheese and red wine for the picnic *cum* seduction, don't be surprised if you hear, "Sorry, honey. I have a headache!" Cheeses with the most pain potential include: Stilton, Camembert, Cheddar, Boursault, Emmenthaler, Gruyere, Roquefort, Brie, Parmesan, Romano, provolone and mozzarella. Even "everyday" varieties like brick, processed cheese foods and spreads can do the trick. Cottage cheese and cream cheese are less likely to offend than aged and ripened cheeses.

Other party and snack favorites are high on the headache list: salted crackers, salted tidbits, ham and salami, cheese dips and salty chips. Ouch! Both the salt and the nitrite additives can do you in. But not right away. It might take twelve hours after eating some salty foods before your head begins to hurt. With so much time separating cause and effect, you might never make an association between the two. (For more on salt, see "Passion and Potency," Chapter 22.)

And you like Chinese food? The MSG (monosodium glutamate) that's often added to season Oriental specialties is the cause of "Chinese Restaurant Syndrome." The intensity of the ensuing headache depends on the ingested dose. If your head always feels like it's in a vice when you've eaten Eastern dishes, make sure you request that the MSG be omitted when your choices from columns A and B are being prepared.

Nuts can do it too. Nuts! These are potentially so powerful that even a few little pieces in a cookie or candy bar can trigger a headache in some sensitive people. Cashews and peanuts are the worst, with coconut close behind. The problem with coconut is that coconut by-products are used in a wide variety of food products and are major ingredients in most cream and whipped-cream substitutes. In his book *Control of Migraine,* John Brainard, M.D., notes that dessert topping can "flatten a susceptible migraine patient for the next 24 hours." And if it's pineapple cream pie then there's real trouble, because pineapple, especially fresh, can compound the problem.

Other foods can do it too. Milk, cream and ice cream may seem soothing to some people. However, they can bring on a headache in a few. Cooked milk (as in custard) does not appear as offensive.

You don't even have to consume any of these ingestibles to get a headache. Not eating can cause one, too. In fact, skipping meals brings on a self-inflicted hypoglycemia (low blood sugar), which can produce symptoms including irritability and headache. The Rx? Food. Even though you think you have a legitimate excuse to avoid eating ("Don't have the time!" "On a diet!")—putting off your stomach will eventually put the bite on your head.

Hypoglycemia is currently in vogue, and a lot of people are pinning their headaches, fatigue and anxiety on it. The causes vary, but the most obvious (skipping meals) should not be overlooked. A few people are "true" hypoglycemics with blood sugar levels plummeting after a glucose tolerance test. Other people have the symptoms without being truly hypoglycemic, although they are sugar-sensitive.

A lot of physicians don't buy the hypoglycemia routine. If you react to sugar, you may not fit the medical model of hypoglycemia. Arguing about what to call it might not be productive. The treatment boils down to regular, frequent meals interspersed with some snacks. Sugar can pull you out of an immediate slump, but it can also put you into another—so avoid sweets. It's wiser to "head it off at the pass" by eating regularly and by substituting fiber foods (fruits, vegetables, whole grains and legumes) for products made with sugar and/or white flour. The presence of fiber usually helps slow down the release of sugar into the bloodstream, creating a kind of "tiny time pill" that delivers tiny amounts of sugar to your bloodstream over a prolonged period of time. This helps eliminate the sugar ups, sugar downs and the sugar blues.

The other happy note about fiber: It prevents constipation. Lots of people with irregularity also complain of headaches. So drink plenty of fluids, get some physical activity and munch on fiber foods to feel good end to end!

If you are dieting, you might be skipping meals or skipping carbohydrates, and either will cause your head to pound. Another diet trick, the high-protein diet, can also cause constipation. In addition, the ketosis (abnormal burning of fat) that occurs on a high-protein diet can further contribute to headache.

If you've misinterpreted the information in this book about vitamin A, you may have started taking huge amounts of it. Taking excessive doses can produce a variety of symptoms including nausea, vomiting, blurring of vision and an intense headache.

Even though it appears that a headache just pops up, it doesn't just happen. There's always a cause. Fortunately, most headaches are not symptomatic of anything too serious. But there is always that possibility. If your headaches are like a bolt out of the blue with a shattering severity, or if they are accompanied by a blurring of vision or a loss of alertness, check with your physician. Also, headaches marked by fever and neck stiffness, as well as those that are recurrent or increase in frequency and/or intensity, can signify a deeper problem. Other problems that can lead to head pain include high blood pressure, injuries, sinus trouble and eye problems. Headaches that are always localized to one specific area should be evaluated.

Though there are a variety of reasons for headaches, what you eat can play a major role in triggering pain between your ears. This is especially true if you are prone to migraines. Some tasty foods are torturous treats for you, proverbial brain blasters! So if you find yourself saying, "Not tonight, honey, I've got a headache," think about *what* you have eaten during the last 24 hours or *if* you have eaten recently. Most likely you'll find a clue. Next time you won't have that headache. . . .

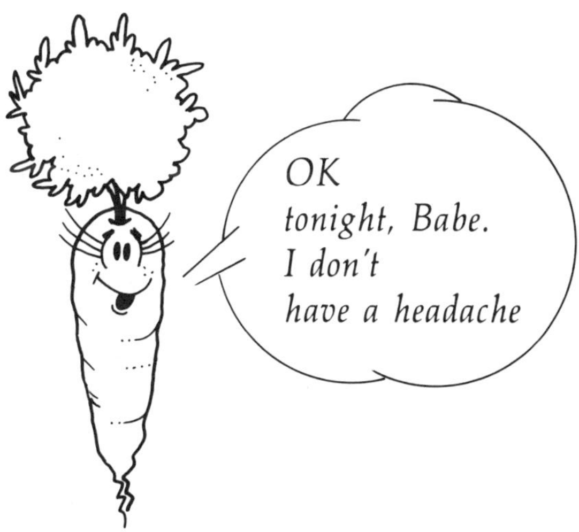

18
TOO TIRED

If your "get up and go" got up and went, leaving you too pooped to come . . . and go as you'd like, then read on. I bet that a lot of things you do to charge yourself up actually wear you down.

Out of energy? Do you reach for sugar? You've already found out that sugar gives you a quick burst of energy. Yet within 90 minutes, the burst often busts. Your blood sugar drops. You droop. Actually, a high-sugar diet may contribute to your tiredness in two ways. First, it may alter the secretion of insulin or other substances involved in blood sugar regulation, producing blood sugar changes. The second is less immediate, but more insidious. Keep reading.

Sugar is a carbohydrate. Like all carbohydrates, its utilization by your body requires the presence of vitamins and minerals. Unlike wholesome carbohydrate-containing foods (whole grains, fruits, vegetables and legumes), sugar supplies none. If you eat a lot of sugar (see "Getting Stoned," Chapter 15) you'll also create a need for more nutrients, especially thiamine (vitamin B-1.) This vitamin is also essential for the health of your nerves and gastrointestinal tract. Not only will a relatively inadequate thiamine supply strip you of stamina, it will also make you depressed, irritable and apathetic. You'll feel fatigued. Too much "sugar bowl" may lead to some bowel disturbances as well. Ah ha! You say. All I have to do is take a vitamin pill to make up. Wrong! Sugar still has other effects, such as its ability to overstimulate insulin, which cannot be "fixed up" by a vitamin pill. (Supplements are meant to do just that: supplement. If you think vitamin/mineral pills are a cover for poor eating habits, you're only kidding—and hurting—yourself!)

Do you down doughnuts, etc., with your coffee? This is a double whammy. Were you aware that caffeine can also stimulate the flow of insulin? Coffee coupled with confections causes your blood sugar to dip. Within an hour and a half or so of this "typical" breakfast, I bet there are a lot of nervous Neals and Nellies out there. That makes me nervous. I'll tell you why:

When blood sugar goes down, coordination also declines.Think of all those people driving cars, planes and trucks out there who've just dunked a doughnut (or the equivalent). It's scary enough to make you drink! But that's no good either. Some British researchers indict noontime gin-and-tonics (drinks mixed with sweet mixers) for causing afternoon traffic accidents. Why? They pin the blame on the low blood sugar that arrives a couple of hours afterwards. I'm sure you've noticed yourself nodding off in the afternoon after a cocktail at lunch. Not only are you sleepy, you're also less coordinated. This is not a great combination for someone who's driving.

The other problem with this blood sugar business is that you become cranky. When you're in an irritable mood, your relationships may not be a sweet as you'd like them to be. So your day at home or the office is a little more difficult. By the time your spouse or lover comes home, there may be wargames, not love play.

You may have heard that some "carbos" at bedtime help you sleep. True! A high-carboydrate meal or snack facilitates the passage of tryptophan, an amino acid, into the brain. In turn, brain chemistry is altered so that you become pleasantly drowsy. Sleep comes easily. Supplements of tryptophan can also be taken with the carbos to induce the sandman. Have a glass of juice, some bread or a muffin before you turn the lights out. Have a bran muffin. That might help you drift off at night and get you "going" in the morning!!

Contrary to granny's advice, a glass of milk at bedtime is not a good soporific. Even though milk is full of tryptophan, it also contains other amino acids that compete with tryptophan for entry into the brain. A high-carbohydrate, low-protein snack does more to elevate brain tryptophan levels than a protein food that's rich in tryptophan!

Alcohol can make you drowsy. Unfortunately, it also ruins a good night's rest by interfering with REM (dream-state) sleep. If you're prone to insomnia, taking a nightcap will probably make your problem worse.

As long as we're looking at this insomnia issue, we shouldn't overlook caffeine. It also interferes with sleep. When you're caffeinated, it may take you longer to fall asleep and/or you might be restless through the night. The other problem with caffeine is that it hypes up your nerves, but does little to waken your muscles. Your body can be tired while your nerves are stimulated. Caffeine can mask fatigue. The longer you put off a decent rest, the more fatigued you'll be.

There's nothing wrong with taking a nap every now and then. A lot of creative people do. Sleep can help you synthesize material. Why stay up all night forcing an issue when you can resolve it during sleep and see it clearly when you wake up? Beats me. (It's time for my nap . . . . No, maybe I'll go for a jog instead.)

Most of us spend more time on our rear ends than our feet. That's just the way things are today. If you're not getting any physical activity other than moving from chair to chair, you're bound to be bushed.

Table 18-1: Foods High in Iron

FOOD	PORTION SIZE	mg IRON PER PORTION
Protein Foods of Animal Origin		
Beef, lean	3 oz	4.0-5.0
Chicken	3 oz	1.0
Egg	1 average	1.0
Fish	3 oz	1.0
Liver	3 oz	7.0-8.0
Pork, lean	3 oz	4.0-5.0
Sardines (in oil)	8 medium	3.5
Protein Foods of Plant Origin:		
Beans (kidney, lima, etc.) cooked	½ cup	2.0-4.0
Lentils, cooked	½ cup	1.5
Tofu	4 oz	2.0-4.0
Cereals and Grains:		
Bagel	1	1.0
Biscuit	1	0.5
Bread, French	1 slice	0.5
Bread, whole-wheat or white	1 slice	0.5-1
Cereals, whole-grain, cooked	1 cup	1.5-2
Pancake	1	0.5
Pasta, white enriched, cooked (macaroni, noodles and spaghetti)	1 cup	1.5
Rice, brown, cooked	1 cup	1.0
Rice, enriched, cooked	1 cup	1.5
Tortilla, corn	1 6″ diameter	1.0
Wheat germ	1 tablespoon	1.0
Fruits:		
Average for those unlisted	½ cup	0.5
Apricots, raw	2-3	0.5
Apricots, dried	4 halves	1.5
Prune juice	½ cup	5.0
Prunes, dried	4 large	2.0
Raisins	2½ tablespoon	1.0
Vegetables:		
Average for those unlisted	½ cup	0.5-1.0
Chard, cooked	3/5 cup	3.0
Dandelion greens, cooked	½ cup	3.0
Mixed vegetables, frozen, cooked	1 cup	2.5
Mustard greens, cooked	½ cup	2.0
Parsley, chopped	2 tablespoons	1.0
Peas, green, cooked	2/3 cup	2.0
Potato, baked	1 small	1.0
Spinach, cooked	½ cup	2.0
Squash, acorn, baked	½	2.0

Table 18-1: Continued (iron content)

FOOD	PORTION SIZE	mg IRON PER PORTION
Squash, butternut, baked	1 cup	1.5
Sweet potato, baked	1 large	1.5
Tomato sauce	1 cup	2.0
Turnip greens, cooked	½ cup	2.0

Cooking in iron pots greatly increases the iron content.

Based on: Pennington, J. B.; Church, H. N. *Bowes and Church's Food Values of Portions Commonly Used*, Philadelphia: J. B. Lippincott, 1980.

Exercise is very invigorating. Find something that you enjoy—walking, bellydancing, crewing, swimming, skiing, cycling, running, and so on. Why not do a variety of activities during any given week? That way you won't get bored. Besides, different activities use different muscles, and that's a plus.

As you can see, what you drink can influence the quality of your sleep. Incidentally, not drinking enough can also tire you out. If you get into heavy-duty sweating with the activities you pursue, you'll tire quickly unless you replenish your water supply (see "Fluid Relationships," Chapter 23.)

What else can make you tired? Why, "tired blood" of course! Although a whole bunch of nutrients are necessary for building blood, the best known one is iron. Not enough dietary iron and you can get iron-deficiency anemia, the so-called tired blood. Iron is necessary for the formation of hemoglobin, the part of the blood that transports oxygen to your cells. Without an adequate O_2 supply, you'll tucker out easily.

You don't have to be anemic to be deficient in iron. You can have a normal hemoglobin reading, because your iron "stores" will be depleted first, and blood levels of iron are the last to go. Anything that stresses your iron supply may suddenly slip you into anemic status. This would include blood loss from illness, injury or donation, pregnancy and prolonged heavy physical workouts, during which you can lose as much as one gram of iron in your sweat.

Women will have a tough time getting all their iron from food. The RDA for menstruating women is 18 mg. Since every well-selected 1,000 calories supplies only 6 mg of iron, you can see why most women don't get enough. How many women eat 3,000 calories a day? Older women, boys and men need less—10 mg. It's easier for them to get what they need. Yet everyone needs to know that certain factors help iron absorption while others hinder it.

First of all, do you get enough? See Table 18-1 and find out. The iron in meats, called heme iron, is the easiest to absorb. The iron from grains and beans is a little less available. The presence of heme iron in a meal makes the other kind (non-heme) more available. Other foods favor iron absorption, too. Take broccoli, orange juice—anything containing vitamin C will do the trick. What's high in vitamin C? (See Table 3-1 in "High-Class Pap," Chapter 3.)

That's the good news. Here's the bad news. Certain factors interfere with the absorption of iron from plant foods. One is phytate, which is found in the outer bran layer of whole grains. When grains are yeast-raised as in bread, however, there seems to be little problem with phytate. Tannin in tea is a big offender. Drinking tea with your meals reduces non-heme iron absorption by 62%. Coffee reduces it by 35%. In contrast orange juice can almost double the amount of iron that's absorbed.

Another anti-anemia agent is folic acid. Unfortunately, folic acid is frequently forgotten. That's easy to do when you skip fresh foods. Remember this line: Foliage for folic acid. The best sources are leafy greens. (For more info on folic acid, see Table 8-1.)

A lot of things can make us tired, including the things we use to perk up.

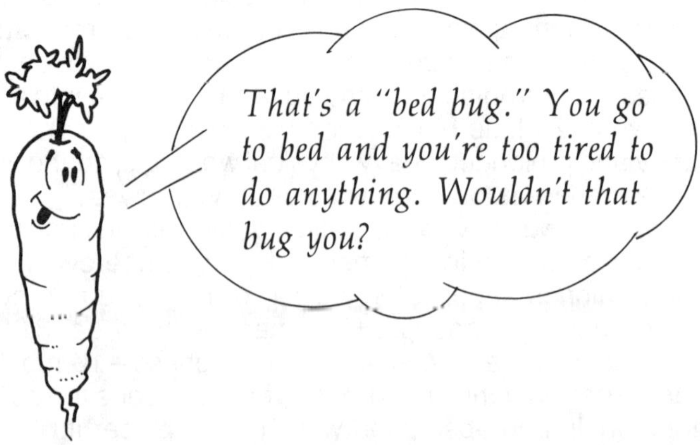

19

FIBER FOR FLUFFIES

Fiber for fluffies? What on earth is a fluffy? A form of natural biofeedback, it's your "end" product of a high fiber diet. When you eat hard—i.e. fiber filled—foods, your stool comes out soft and "fluffy." When you eat soft foods — i.e. fiber-free — foods, your stool comes out hard. (The famous British surgeon who rediscovered fiber, Dr. Denis Burkitt, once summarized this food philosophy by saying "hard in, soft out.")

Fiber is the indigestible part of plants, and it plays a crucial role in your "solid waste disposal system." In this regard, fiber does two things. First, it stimulates peristalsis (the rhythmic contractions of your intestine). This enables waste materials to move through your gut faster. Second, it has an amazing ability to hold on to water. This means that you get large, soft (yet formed), "fluffy" bowel movements that are easy to pass. Fluffy, frequent stools are your hedge against the heartbreak of constipation as well as the more serious condition of diverticulosis. You don't have to strain to make a "fluffy," and that's a real plus! Straining to "do your thing" increases your chances of developing hemorrhoids.

Fiber's ability to make your movements fluffy and frequent is directly tied to its role in preventing colon cancer. First of all, a fluffy stool essentially dilutes the concentration of any toxic substances that may be in your BM. Besides, fiber causes its efficient and quick removal, leaving little time for any harmful substance to adversely affect the bowel lining. (At this time, it seems that excessive fat consumption contributes some harmful substances to the ol' waste material! Not to worry! When you increase your fiber foods, you'll automatically reduce the fat content of your diet!)

Fiber does a lot more for you, too. It can help you stay (or get) slim. Fiber foods are bulky and, by the spoonful, are dramatically lower in calories than foods high in fat. Fiber foods fill you up before you get filled out. On the other hand, foods high in fat pack an astronomical amount of calories into small spaces. A small cube (an inch or so) of fudge and a large apple (about 3" in diameter) each contain approximately 125 calories. A certain friend of mine (whose name will be witheld to protect the guilty) thinks nothing of eating several pieces of fudge after dinner. Give her an apple and she can barely eat half. Fiber-depleted foods are just too easy to eat; they fill you out, not up.

Sugar is among the most compact and fiberless carbohydrates around. To make one teaspoonful of the stuff, you have to process a sugar beet as large as a grapefruit. Yet the sugar and the beet have the same caloric content! With the calories removed from its original fibrous source, sugar ranks high on the soft foods list. It's hard to imagine that the average American eats 12 tablespoons of sugar a day. Incredible? Yes! Impossible? No! You probably don't use a lot of sugar from your sugar bowl, but many of the food products you eat might contain a hefty portion of it. (For a list, see Table 15-1 in "Getting Stoned," Chapter 15.) If you've ever had four cans of soda on a hot summer's day, you've done it. If you were to get all that sugar from its original source, you would have to eat a sugar beet the size of a big head!

Sugar is rapidly absorbed into your bloodstream. At first your blood sugar level rises quite a bit above normal. However, sugar also overstimulates the secretion of insulin, which then pushes your blood sugar down to fairly low levels. So you feel tired. Some people mistakenly reach for more sugar to get pepped up. Ultimately just the reverse happens—too much sugar can make you feel tired! (For more on being tired, see "Too Tired," Chapter 18.)

Even though starches are eventually broken down to glucose, or blood sugar, the presence of fiber in a food usually delays the absorption of glucose. In essence, many fiber foods (especially beans & oats) provide you with a steady supply of energy over a long period of time. Unlike sugary foods, some fiber foods do not tax your insulin reserves. Think of fiber foods as another kind of those "tiny time pills"—this one delivering a relatively long-lasting and steady supply of energy to your bloodstream. Sugar, on the other hand, gives you a brief high, and shortly thereafter drives your blood sugar quickly into "the pits." This is why high-fiber diets are currently recommended for diabetics and people with hypoglycemia (low blood sugar). In general, many fiber-rich foods don't demand much insulin, nor do they drive your blood sugar crazy!

Fiber also is protective against heart disease. Because fiber promotes the rapid passage of food and waste through your intestines, less time is available for the absorption of cholesterol. In addition, one class of fiber (soluble fiber including pectin), binds up with some of the fat and cholesterol you've eaten. So less fat and cholesterol are absorbed; instead, some gets shipped out with Number Two. (Note: Pectin is found in apples, citrus fruits, carrots

Table 19-1: Fiber Foods

Fiber is derived only from plant foods. This means that dairy products, eggs, meat, poultry and fish don't provide any. Neither do fats, including butter, margarine, oil, mayonnaise and salad dressings. Sugar, honey and alcohol are also devoid of fiber.

FOOD	PORTION SIZE	gms FIBER PER PORTION
Legumes:		
Beans, brown, cooked	½ cup	8.4
Beans, kidney, cooked	½ cup	9.7
Beans, lima, cooked	½ cup	8.3
Beans, pinto, cooked	½ cup	8.9
Beans, white, cooked	½ cup	7.9
Lentils, cooked	½ cup	3.7
Breads:		
Bran-muffin (whole wheat)	1 average	2.3
Cornbread	1 average square	1.1
French	1 slice	0.7
Pumpernickel	1 slice	1.8
Rye	1 slice	0.8
Sourdough	1 slice	0.7
White	1 slice	0.7
Whole meal (heavy-duty!)	1 slice	2.1
Whole-wheat	1 slice	1.3
Cereals:		
100% Bran	½ cup	4.0
All Bran	1/3 cup	8.4
Bran Chex	½ cup	4.1
Bran, miller's	2 tablespoons	3.5
Corn Chex	¾ cup	2.6
Corn Bran	½ cup	4.4
Corn Flakes	¾ cup	2.6
Fruit n' Fiber	½ cup	3.5
Grapenut Flakes	2/3 cup	2.5
Grapenuts	3 tablespoons	2.7
Oat Bran, dry	¼ cup	5.3
Oat flakes	½ cup	2.5
Oatmeal, instant, dry	1 package	3.3
Oats, whole, dry	1/3 cup	3.8
Post Toasties	1 cup	2.5
Puffed Wheat	¾ cup	3.4
Oatmeal, rolled, cooked	1 cup	3.2
Ralston, dry	3 tablespoons	2.1
Shredded wheat	1 biscuit	2.8
Shredded Wheat, spoon size	1 oz	4.4
Total	¾ cup	2.5
Wheaties	¾ cup	2.6
Wheatina, cooked	2/3 cup	2.2

Table 19-1 Continued (fiber content)

FOOD	PORTION SIZE	gms FIBER PER PORTION
Crackers:		
Graham	2 squares	1.4
Ry-Krisp	3 wafers	2.3
Saltines	6 crackers	0.8
Triscuits	2 crackers	2.0
Wheat Thins	6 crackers	2.2
Fruits:		
Apple, fresh or cooked	1 large	4.0
Apricots	2	1.4
Banana	1 mediuim	3.0
Blackberries	¾ cup	6.7
Cherries	10 large	1.1
Fig, dried	1 medium	3.7
Grapefruit	½	0.8
Grapes, black, fresh	15	0.5
Grapes, white, fresh	10	0.5
Melon, canteloupe	1 cup	1.6
Melon, honeydew	1 cup	1.5
Melon, watermelon	1 cup	1.4
Nectarine, raw	1 small	1.5
Orange	1 small	1.6
Peach, fresh	1 medium	2.3
Pear, fresh	½ medium	2.0
Pineapple	½ cup	0.8
Plum, fresh	3 small	1.8
Prunes, dried	2	2.8
Raisins	3 tablespoons	2.0
Raspberries, red, fresh	1 cup	9.2
Strawberries, fresh	1 cup	3.1
Tangerine	1 large	2.0
Grains:		
Buckwheat groats (Kasha), cooked	1 cup	9.0
Bulgur, cooked	1 cup	9.0
Popcorn, popped	3 cups	3.0
Rice, brown, cooked	1 cup	4.8
Rice, white, cooked	1 cup	1.5
Nuts:		
Almonds, shelled	2 tablespoons or ½ oz	2.2
Peanuts, roasted	1 tablespoon	0.8
Peanut butter	2 tablespoons	3.0
Pecans	1 tablespoon	0.5
Walnuts	1 tablespoon	1.1

Table 19-1 Continued (fiber content)

FOOD	PORTION SIZE	gms FIBER PER PORTION
Pasta:		
Macaroni, cooked	½ cup	0.6
Macaroni, whole wheat, cooked	½ cup	2.8
Noodles, whole wheat, cooked	½ cup	2.8
Spaghetti, cooked	½ cup	0.8
Spaghetti, whole-wheat, cooked	½ cup	2.8
Vegetables:		
Asparagus	½ cup	3.5
Bean sprouts	½ cup	1.5
Beans, green, cooked	½ cup	2.1
Beets, cooked	½ cup	2.1
Broccoli, cooked	½ cup	3.5
Brussels sprouts, cooked	½ cup	2.3
Cabbage, white, cooked	½ cup	2.1
Carrots, raw	½ cup	1.8
Cauliflower, cooked	½ cup	1.6
Celery, raw	½ cup	1.1
Corn, sweet, fresh	1 medium ear	5.2
Cucumber, raw	½ cup	1.1
Eggplant, raw	½ cup	2.5
Kale, cooked	½ cup	1.3
Lettuce, fresh	1 cup	0.8
Mushrooms, raw	½ cup	0.9
Mustard greens, raw	1 cup	2.0
Okra, raw	½ cup	1.6
Onion, raw	½ cup	1.2
Peas, green, cooked	½ cup	6.7
Pepper, green, raw	½ cup	1.1
Potato, sweet, cooked	½ medium	2.1
Potato, white, baked	1 medium	3.8
Radishes, raw	½ cup	1.3
Spinach, fresh	1 cup	0.2
Squash, summer, cooked	½ cup	2.0
Squash, winter, cooked	1 cup	7.0
Tomato, cooked	½ cup	1.5
Tomato, raw	1 medium	1.5
Turnip, cooked	½ cup	2.0
Yam, cooked	½ cup	2.6
Zucchini, raw	½ cup	2.0

Adapted from:
Anderson, J. W. *Diabetes*. New York: Arco Publishing, Inc., 1981.
Burkitt, D. *Eat Right To Stay Healthy and Enjoy Life More.* New York: Arco Publishers, Inc., 1979.

Figure 19-1

FIBER FOR FLUFFIES!

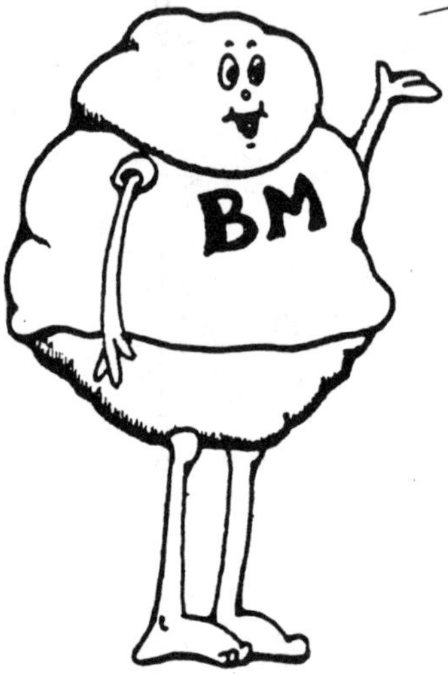

Hi there! For me, you must eat carbohydrate foods of the unrefined variety. Whole-wheat and whole-grain breads are high in fiber. So are whole-grain cereals like oatmeal, wheat flakes, shredded wheat, bran cereals, unprocessed bran and brown rice.

Popcorn is a neat high-fiber snack.

Make sure you eat a lot of fresh fruits and fresh vegetables that are raw or very lightly steamed. Dried fruits such as prunes and raisins are good too.

Legumes (dried peas, beans, lentils) are also high in fiber and can be used as meat substitutes.

This hardened little fellow is a sinker. Sinkers happen when you eat carbohydrate foods that have been refined like white bread, English muffins, soda crackers, and refined cereals such as farina, cream of wheat, corn flakes, rice krispies and sweetened "children's cereals."

Cookies, candies, soda pop, cakes, pies and donuts are made with white flour and sugar. They are high in calories but low in fiber.

Following a high-protein, low-carbohydrate diet will also produce sinkers because hardly any fibrous fruits, vegetables or grains are eaten.

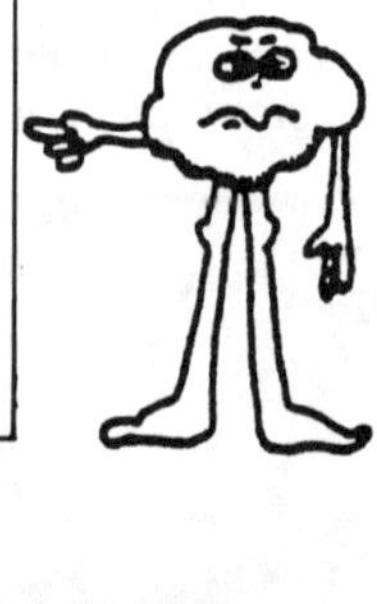

and other root vegetables.) Oat bran (found in oatmeal) and legumes also contain soluble fibers that exert a protective effect on heart health.

The protective action of fiber foods is a result of the presence of fiber per se, as well as the fact that these foods tend to be loaded with vitamins and minerals and other protective substances such as "indoles." Found in members of the cabbage-cauliflower-broccoli-rutabaga family, indoles have some anticancer properties. So it's important to eat a variety of fruits, vegetables, whole grains and legumes to get everything fiber foods have to offer. Simply adding bran to a high-fat, high-sugar diet is not good enough.

See Table 19-1 to find out about the fiber content of foods. A recent article in *The Lancet*, a British medical journal, noted that a fiber intake of 37 grams/day appeared to be protective against death from chronic diseases, including cancer and heart disease. As mentioned previously, vegetarians eating 28 grams of fiber had a lower cancer risk than omnivorous types eating 12 grams. Most of us would do well to boost our fiber intakes up to 25-50 grams per day. So check out the chart. How do you know if you are getting enough fiber? The bottom line is that the easiest way to relate to fiber is to see its effect on your bowel habits. Get some biofeedback: Check your stool. Is it a fluffy? (See Fig. 19-1)

Several years after I introduced "fluffies" to a group of top-level execs, I ran into one of them who said, "Candy, I have been thinking about you every day now!"

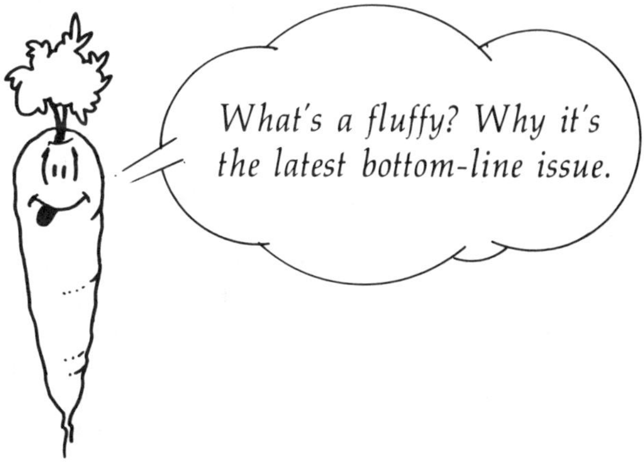
What's a fluffy? Why it's
the latest bottom-line issue.

20

STRIP AND UNDRESS

It's no surprise that sex is better when you strip and undress. In fact, it's true on two accounts. The first is obvious. You might have some trouble identifying the second, however: trimming the fat from your fare. As we've already discussed, your risk of hormone-dependent cancers (breast, prostate) goes up as you fork up more fat. To keep your sexy parts in good condition, strip that fat off your meat and undress your salads!

Salad dressing is subversive. Just when you think you've been "good" by dishing up a huge plate of rabbit food, you can "blow it" by covering it with a thick layer of dressing. Typical toppings total 200-300 calories per 1/4 cup (average salad bar ladle). And it's virtually all fat! Next time you're at a salad bar, watch the folks ladle up. Very few stop at one! Some people use four—nearly 1,000 calories of the stuff! (Salads aren't fattening, right?) Eating a totally naked salad might be tough if you're the type who smothers greens with dressing, but you can cut down on how much you use. If you're a two-ladle type, use one. You can always stretch creamy dressings with buttermilk, yogurt or blended cottage cheese. Adding a bit more vinegar, a pinch of sugar and some water will do the same for the oil and vinegar variety. Some people like plain rice vinegar or malt vinegar on their salads. Why not try it yourself? There's always a squeeze of fresh lemon to add some zip. You might even like your salads totally undressed!

Whether or not "real men" eat quiche is debatable. One thing quiche-eaters should know is that the genuine quiche, a rich custard of cream and cheese nestled in a pastry crust, probably contains 45-50 grams of fat per piece! That's all the fat most people need per day!

By now you are probably well aware that red meats contain quite a bit of fat. However, some cuts are fairly lean. That's why you need to shop in the "tenderloin district" of your market—beef and pork tenderloin are almost free of marbling and much lower in fat than a steak. Your average steakhouse dinner of steak, "loaded" spud, salad (no doubt heavily dressed) and bread and butter contains a huge lard load: Over 50% of its calories come from fat!

It doesn't have to be fancy to be fat-filled. Fast foods are also high in fat, with typical meals tipping to the 50%-calories-as-fat range. The special gigunda-burga at these places runs high in fat. So do the chicken and fish-wiches as well. Yes, I know you've heard that chicken and fish are low in fat. They are—until you bread them and drop them into the deepfat fryer. Of all the entree selections available, the lowly hamburger happens to be lowest in fat.

Do you like to nibble on cheese before dinner? Cheese is nutritious, but it is high in fat. It's great added to a vegetarian casserole or slipped between two slices of whole wheat for a luncheon sandwich, but is not the best prelude to a meal that's most likely already high in fat.

If you think that desserts are mostly sugar, you'll be surprised to learn that some of your favorites are also high in fat. My favorite is! I love that Häagen-Dazs! One reason why it tastes so good is that it's twice as rich as most other ice creams. (I eat nude salads to compensate!) Cheesecake, carrot cake, cookies,—they are all fairly high in fat. That makes them special treats, but not daily bread.

One thing that bugs me about fat is that it doesn't take up much space. You can get a substantial amount of calories from relatively small volumes of it without getting filled up. For instance, a tablespoon of butter has as many calories as the potato you put it on. How many people stop at one tablespoon of butter? Yet most people stop at one potato! A half cup of rich ice cream has as many calories as four big apples. You might go for two scoops of ice cream. It's doubtful you'd even eat two apples in a row. Fats fill you out before they fill you up.

Nuts are a nemesis worthy of note. Any nut already out of its shell is, in effect, a refined food. If the shell were on all the nuts you eat, chances are you'd eat a lot fewer nuts. Why? It's hard work breaking those buggers out of their shells, and then you have to clean up the mess afterwards. Nuts that are already shelled are very easy to eat. A 5½-oz. can of peanuts contains 850 calories. That dinky packet you get on an airplane contains about 100. Nuts are tasty and crunchy and provide some vitamin E. Stop at a handful, not a can-full.

Our national fat intake currently accounts for a whopping 40% of our calories, and at that level we're at high risk for cancer and heart disease. Cutting that to 20-30% would bring your fat intake more in line with levels associated with a lower risk of these two diseases—but since some fat is essential, don't cut it all out completely.

Take the time to figure out how much fat you typically eat by using Table 20-1. As you go through the list, circle or highlight your favorites. In addition, look at other foods you are also fond of, but which have a lower fat content. If it turns out that your fat intake is high, then make a decision about eating fewer fatty foods. You can do

Table 20-1: Figuring Fat From Your Fare

To determine how many of your calories come from fat you need to know how many calories you usually eat each day. If you haven't the slightest idea, here are some "average" figures for you to use.

CALORIES/DAY

Women:	12-17:	1800	Men:	12-17:	2600	Yours: ______
	18-44:	1600		18-54:	2400	
	45+	1400		55+:	2000	

FAT/DAY

In the FAT IN YOUR FARE table, the fat content of foods is given in grams. Each gram (gm) of fat yields 9 calories. Use the reference below to see how many grams of fat/day equals 20-30% of your total caloric intake.*

AVERAGE CALORIC INTAKE	PERCENT OF CALORIES FROM FAT 20%	30%	40%
1200	27 gm	40 gm	53 gm
1400	31	47	62
1500	33	50	67
1600	36	53	71
1800	40	60	80
2000	44	67	89
2200	49	73	98
2400	53	80	107
2600	58	87	116
3000	66	100	133

An ideal intake would be in the 20-30% range. What's your ideal fat intake? ______ grams

How does your actual fat consumption compare? See FAT IN YOUR FARE

FAT IN YOUR FARE

FOOD	SERVING SIZE	GRAMS OF FAT
Bread/Grains:		
Bagel	1 whole	2
Banana or fruit bread	1 slice	2
Bread	1 slice	½
Biscuit	2″ diameter	5
Cereals, except granola	1 oz	1
Cornbread	2″ × 2″ × 1	5
Crackers, buttery (Ritz, Triscuits)	5	5
Croissant	1 small	6
Danish	1 small	7
French toast	1 slice	5
Granola	¼ cup	5
Granola bar	1	5
Hot dog/Burger bun	1 whole	2
Muffin, plain	1 (2″ diameter)	5

*Adapted from: Liebman, B. "Ferreting Fat from Your Diet." *Nutrition Action*, 1982, 9, 12-13.

Table 20-1 Continued (Fat)

FAT IN YOUR FARE FOOD	SERVING SIZE	GRAMS OF FAT
Noodles, plain	1 cup, cooked	½
Noodles, egg	1 cup, cooked	2
Oatmeal	1 cup, cooked	3
Pancake	5″ in diameter	5
Pasta	1 cup, cooked	½
Patty shell (pastry)	1	18
Popcorn, popped with oil (no butter added!)	1½ cups	1
Potatoes, french fried	8 (each 2″ × 3½″)	10
Potato or corn chips	1 oz	10
Pretzels	1 oz	1
Rice	1 cup, cooked	negligible
Tortilla, corn or flour	6″ in diameter	½
Waffle, homemade	1 medium	8
Waffle, frozen	1 medium	3
Dairy Products:		
Cheese, cottage, low fat	½ cup	2
Cheese, cottage, creamed	½ cup	5
Cheese, mozzarella, ricotta farmer's, neufchatel	1 oz	4
Cheese, cheddar-type	1 oz	8
Cheese, parmesan	3 tablespoons	5
Ice cream	½ cup	10
Ice Cream (rich)	½ cup	18
Ice milk	½ cup	2
Milk, skim	1 cup	0
Milk, 1%	1 cup	1
Milk, 2% (low fat)	1 cup	5
Milk, whole	1 cup	8
Yogurt, low-fat	1 cup	5
Yogurt, whole	1 cup	8
Meat, Chicken & Seafood:		
Beef (chipped, chuck, flank tenderloin, round, sirloin, heart)	1 oz	3
Beef, ground (15% fat)	1 oz	6
Beef, ground (20+% fat)	1 oz	8
Beef (corned, rib eye)	1 oz	6
Beef (steaks—club, rib)	1 oz	8
Cold Cuts	1 oz	8
Egg	1	6
Fish, fresh or frozen "white" fish	1 oz	1
Fish (salmon, rainbow trout)	1 oz	4
Fish (sardines, drained)	3	3
Fish (shellfish—clams, crab, lobsters		

Table 20-1 Continued (Fat)

FAT IN YOUR FARE FOOD	SERVING SIZE	GRAMS OF FAT
shrimp, oysters, scallops)	1 oz	1
Fish (tuna in oil)	¼ cup	4
Fish (tuna in water)	¼ cup	1/5
Frankfurter	1 average	10
Lamb (leg, rib, sirloin, shank, shoulders)	1 oz	3
Organ meats (liver, kidney sweetbreads)	1 oz	3
Pork (bacon)	2 slices	8
Pork (leg, ham, smoked)	1 oz	3
Pork (shoulder, Boston butt)	1 oz	6
Pork (spareribs, loin, ground, devilled ham)	1 oz	8
Poultry (chicken, turkey without skin)	1 oz	1
Poultry (chicken, turkey with skin)	1 oz	2
Poultry (chicken, fried)	1 oz	5
Poultry (capon, duck, goose)	1 oz	8
Veal (all cuts, except breast)	1 oz	3
Veal breast	1 oz	7
Veal cutlet, fried	1 oz	4
Legumes, Nuts, Seeds:		
Beans, cooked	1 cup	1
Beans (soybeans, cooked)	1 cup	5
Beans (soybeans curd Tofu)	3½ oz	4
Soybean milk	1 cup	4
Almonds	10 whole	5
Nuts	6 small	5
Pecans	2 large whole	5
Peanuts, Spanish	20 whole	5
Peanuts, Virginia	10 whole	5
Peanut butter	1 tablespoon	8
Walnuts	4-5 halves	5
Seeds	1 tablespoon	5
Fruits, Vegetables:		
Avocado	½	19
Fruit (fresh fruits & juices)	½ cup	Negligible
Vegetables, fresh or frozen without butter/sauce	½ cup	Negligible
Fast Foods:		
Burger, cheese	1	13
Burger, plain	1	9
Burger, special (Whopper, Big Mac)	1	32
Chicken, fried	1 dinner pack chicken only	46 18

Table 20-1 Continued (Fat)

FAT IN YOUR FARE FOOD	SERVING SIZE	GRAMS OF FAT
Chicken, fried, x-tra crispy	1 dinner pack	54
	chicken only	21
Fish, Whaler	1	46
Fish, Fillet o'Fish	1	23
Fish, fried (no chips)	1 serving	20
Pizza, Pizza Hut	1 slice	6
Shake	1 average	10
Sweets:		
Cake (no icing)	3″ × 3″ × 2″	8
Cake (with icing)	3″ × 3″ × 2″	18
Cheesecake	1/9 of 9″ cake	35
Cookie	1 average	3
Pie, fruit or cream	1/6 of 9″ pie	18
Pie, pecan	1/6 of 9″ pie	35
Sherbert	½ cup	5
Fats, Oils, Spreads, Dressings:		
Butter	1 teaspoon	4
Cream, heavy, whipping	1 tablespoon	5
Cream, light (half & half)	2 tablespoons	5
Cream, sour	2 tablespoons	5
Cream cheese	2 tablespoons	10
Margarine	1 teaspoon	4
Mayonnaise	1 teaspoon	4
Mayonnaise, low-calorie	1 teaspoon	2
Oil	1 teaspoon	5
Salad dressing, creamy style	1 tablespoon	7
Salad dressing, oil & vinegar	1 tablespoon	5

Figures from: Pennington, J. A.; Church, H. N. *Bowes and Church's Food Values of Portions Commonly Used.* Philadelphia: J. B. Lippincott Company, 1980.
Cumming, C.; Newman, V. *Eater's Guide: Nutrition Basics for Busy People.* Englewood Cliffs: Prentice-Hall, Inc., 1981.
Liebman, B. "Ferreting Fat from Your Diet." *Nutrition Action*, 1982, 9, 12-13.

this by 1) limiting the quantity each time you have some; or 2) by eating it less frequently; or 3) by doing both of the above.

Suppose you realize that T-bones are doing you in. If you want to cut down on fat, it might be tough to give up meat completely. So here's an idea for you:

First step: cut down on the portion size. If you're into 8-12-oz. portions, cut them in half.

Second step: Switch to a leaner cut, e.g., sirloin or tenderloin.

Third step: Rather than eating beef six times a week, eat it three times, and substitute lower-fat alternatives like poultry, fish or a bean-based dish for the rest of your meals.

You might be a revolutionary and able to overthrow old eating habits overnight. Then again, it might take you several months to evolve into a new eating pattern. But I'll bet that by this time next year, you won't want to eat T-bones every day!

Take the time to jot down several ways you can reduce the amount of fat you eat:

____

____

____

____

____

____

Butter, margarine and mayonnaise are all high in fat, so . . .

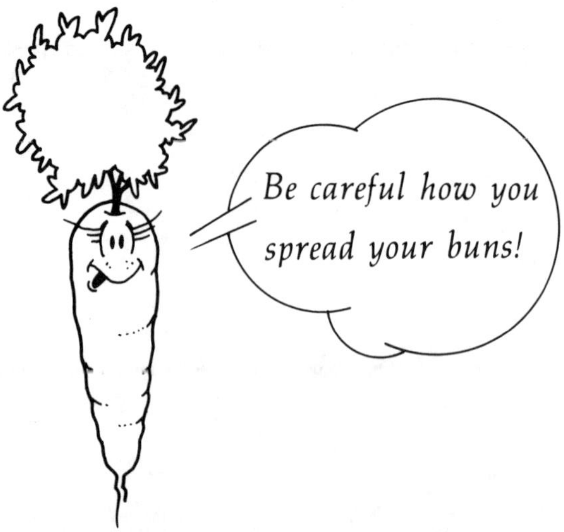

21

TAKE IT OFF

Most people would agree that they feel sexier when they're not flabbier. There are a lot of serious reasons for losing flab: Maintaining a more nearly ideal figure/physique can reduce risk of breast and prostate cancer, and of endometrial cancer as well. Furthermore, the possibility of getting heart disease, maturity-onset diabetes, gallbladder troubles, menstrual abnormalities and high blood pressure goes down as your fat-mass approaches its ideal level. However, the most captivating reason to "take it off" is generally a desire for greater physical attractiveness.

How can you tell if you're fat? Here's the easiest way: The next time you're standing in front of a mirror, open your eyes and take a good look. Jump up and down. The stuff that jiggles is fat. Or else try this: Grab your midsection and give it a pinch. If you've got more than an inch to pinch, you've got some lard to lose. That's the point—it's the excess lard that needs to go.

A lot of people confuse weight with fat. All fat has weight, but not all weight is fat. Getting on a scale tells you how much you weigh, not how fat you are. Some relatively slender-looking people have a fair amount of fat. Some huskier, athletic types are large, but they're lean. What you need to lose is excess fat.

Take the classic example of the college jock turned business executive. Team workouts give way to business lunches and a packed schedule that leaves no time for exercise. His weight never changes. However, his once-sleek triangle physique is now inverted: A muscular upper body slowly disappears as a fat belly develops. The slow metamorphosis from lean to fat takes place as caloric intake remains high and activity patterns fall off. Even people whose weight is fine can be fat if they are physically inactive.

If you found fat, what are you going to do? Run right out to get the latest fad diet in this month's magazines? Run (or walk) out, but forget the magazine. Barring individual differences in such things as metabolism, most of our extra fat comes from what you might call simple inertia. Physical activity has a profound effect on your ability to change flab to firm, and it does it in a variety of ways.

First of all, a moderate amount of activity actually helps curb the ol' appetite. Without some action, we tend to eat more calories than we need. And surprisingly, fat people often eat less than thin people do. The trouble is that fat people eat a lot relative to their requirements: they do not necessarily eat a lot in absolute terms.

Exercise uses up energy. In fact, an hour's worth of jogging (or some wild disco dancing) can increase your day's energy expenditure by 33%! Let's look at a few averages: When an average man, who weighs an average of 150 pounds, engages in an average day's activity, he uses an average of 12 calories per hour. That means he needs 1,800 calories/day. If he goes for an hour's jog and covers an average of six miles, he'll burn off an average of 600 calories. That means to maintain his weight he now needs 2,400 calories. If he keeps his calories at 1,800, he'll lose a little more than a pound of fat per week.

If you don't want to go out and run six miles, try walking a brisk two-or-three miles a day at least five days a week. That's enough to help you shed 10-20 pounds of body fat during the coming year. To keep that fat from forming again, you need to keep moving regularly.

Exercise uses up calories while you *don't* do it. Get this: Regular (daily) physical activity helps increase your metabolic rate so that you burn off more calories even after you've finished exercising. What a deal!

Exercise, as you know, builds up muscle tissue. Within those muscles are little power-houses called mitochondria, which are basically sub-cellular motors. Mitochondria use energy—more muscle, more mitochondria, more energy used up. On the other hand, fat is just a storage depot, or a lot of walks waiting to be taken. Your body is designed to move. Eons back, our forebears needed to move about as they searched for food. When there was no food to be had, they kept their activity to a minimum. Their metabolic rate decreased. Their ability to hold on to fat increased. One theory on overweight suggests that the body still equates inactivity with food scarcity. This wonderful adaptation for survival has outlived its usefulness (at least for the time being). When you have an inactive body that's capable of enhanced fat storage, you're bound to have a weight problem. However, a little physical activity (like a brisk, 45-minute walk every day) can take you out of that calorie-conserving survival mode.

As you can see, fat is easier to lose when you're fit. So don't *have* a fit about being fat—*become* fit and you won't be fat! The added benefit of exercising regularly is that it has a calming effect, a real boon to those who eat whenever they're under stress. Since severe dieting can be very stressful, it can eventually lead to overeating! On the other hand, when you exercise within your physical limits you'll always come back refreshed. You feel so good, you want to get more.

Which cycle would you rather be on?

When it comes to reducing your caloric intake, be careful, because if you eat too little you'll increase your capacity to gain weight! Though it sounds like a contradiction, it's true. You see, your body doesn't know the difference between dieting and starvation. Thus when you diet severely, your body perceives starvation and goes into survival mode. Your metabolic rate goes down. You can get by on much less, but when you increase your caloric intake at the end of your diet, chances are you'll gain weight back very quickly. Strict dieting is counterproductive. Ultimately it makes fat easier to gain, not lose!

Foods full of sugar and/or fat are likely to make you plump up. That's obvious; they're full of calories. But there's more to it than that. Consider our ancestors, who had to work hard to eat, but who ate richer foods during feast time than they normally did. With all that rich food around, they had a temporary increase in appetite, ate more and consequently stored more fat. This "feast-time" increase in appetite is a handy adaptation—if there's a famine around the corner. Even laboratory animals have an increase in appetite when exposed to the "sweet and greasies" compared with times when they get their normal chow. Rich foods increase appetites. More is eaten. More fat gets stored. Boom! Fat in the "boom-boom!" The problem in America is that we feast on rich foods daily, and the famine is (for the present) completely out of sight.

That's why it's a good idea to keep healthful foods around the house. Rather than bringing in a dozen cheesecakes and then having to use your willpower to resist them, leave them at the store. Having "goodies" in your immediate environment is a stressful situation, and what do *you* do when you're stressed? Eat? Also, goodies tend to make us hungry for them, and we respond by eating them up. By keeping the healthful foods around, you are actually doing a little "environmental engineering." You surround yourself with what it takes to lose fat. Makes sense, doesn't it? Plan what you'll bring home from the store. You may have heard that weight control "starts with the cart." I look at it this way: Plan ahead so you don't get more "behind!"

If you want to shed fat, the simplest way to handle eating is to select foods that promote good health and weight control, as in the suggestions given throughout this book. Fasting and severe dieting are out because they do neither. Also eliminated are bizarre diets where you eat a few special foods to the exclusion of all others (high-protein diets, low-carbohydrate diet, all fruit diets, etc). Steer clear of people who want to shoot off your fat with shots, or give you special pills. Look with suspicion at any program that offers miracle cures, or else promises to melt off pounds within a few days.

This last one is really important. Anytime you lose weight faster than two pounds (or three pounds, maximum) per week, you'll be losing water and muscle tissue. You lose a lot of weight, but comparatively little fat. You lose your energy-burning muscle tissue, but keep a considerable amount of your adipose! That's a bad deal. If fat were that easy to melt away, just think of all the grease that would ooze out of your tush and thighs every time you got near a hot stove!

Another decisive fatness factor is your emotions. If you find yourself eating for emotional reasons such as frustration or anger, then you'll not lose your fat until you come to grips with them. Be aware, though, that poor eating habits and a lack of physical activity interfere with your ability to cope. People with a lot of pent-up negative energy are not very sexy, either. Tilt the odds in your own favor—the path to mental well-being includes exercise and a good selection of healthful foods that are low in fat and high in fiber.

There's a food-love relationship that needs to be discussed. You know, food = love. A lot of us learned this one early in the game at home. It goes something like, "If you don't eat my Beef Wellington, you don't love me." You may have gone along expressing your acceptance of grandma (whomever) by accepting every huge morsel (tasty or not). If that's the case, you'll have to find other ways to let that person know how much he or she means to you. With an extra hug and a little extra reassurance of your caring, you can get away with being different at mealtimes.

By the same token, if you're at a loss for words when it comes to telling people how much you love them and you use food as a symbol of your love, try changing the kinds of foods you offer. Better yet, become comfortable in expressing your feelings. Just about everyone loves to hear they're loved. It's a kind of nurturing we all need.

No matter how you slice it, food does mean love. Nurturing and loving are so intertwined that it's hard to separate them. Breaking bread together *is* symbolic. Besides, you eat with your lover more often than you make love together. A lot of positive feeling can be exchanged as you share a meal with your lover, family or friends. The important part is the sharing of self. The kinds of foods you share can still be exquisitely gourmet or plebian, whatever suits the occasion. It's also very possible to have them be low in fat and high in fiber at the same time. (Ask my husband. We certainly have high-fiber meals. He says that living with me has been a very moving experience!) (And for that he's grateful!)

(For a few hints on shortcut ways to take it off, see Table 21-1 and follow the suggestions throughout this book. If you want more info on exercise and other aspects of weight control, check out the resource section. And who knows—you might feel more inclined to get it on as you take it off!)

Incidentally, don't overlook the value of an active sex life in helping you shape up. Just three kisses a day and two amorous interludes

Table 21-1: Short Steps to Shedding Flab

1. Eat early during the day. Have a relatively light dinner in the evening.
2. Drink liquids that are non-caloric. Save calories for foods that fill you up.
3. Drink alcohol in moderation, if at all. Not only is booze big on calories, it may also cause you to lose control around food.
4. Nibble on raw veggies instead of cheese, crackers and nuts.
5. Make sure your meat portions are adequate, not gigantic. A 2-3-oz. portion for a woman or a 3-4-oz. portion for a man is perfect for a meal.
6. Dress salads lightly or leave them naked. Use other fats sparingly as well.
7. Prepare some fresh fruit for dessert. Treat yourself to a favorite dessert once a week.
8. Enjoy some form of physical activity every day.

a week, say some Italian researchers, can result in a nine-pound weight loss during a year's time. Depending on your ardor and its intensity, a kiss burns off 6-12 calories and an interlude of lovemaking, 125-300 calories. Assuming you don't take any vacations, your yearly caloric expenditure would look something like this:

3 average kisses @ 9 calories/kiss × 365 days/year = 9,855 calories
2 amorous interludes @ 212.5 calories each × 52 weeks/year = 22,100 calories

That adds up to a loving 31,955 calories burned off each year. Considering that you need to expend 3,500 calories to lose one pound, that amount of love play may help you kiss off nine pounds annually!

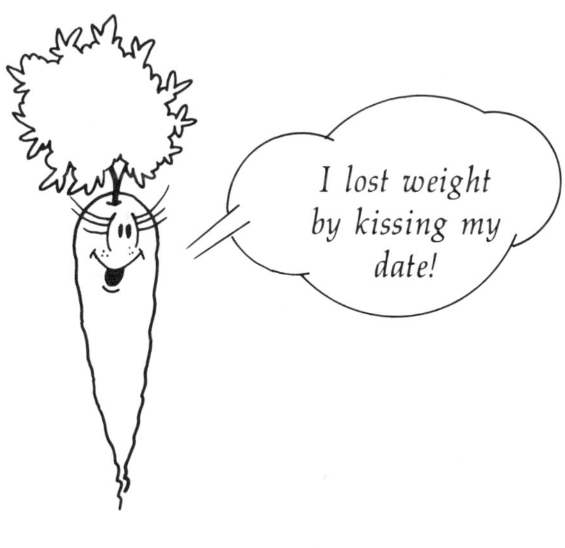

22

PASSION AND POTENCY

What do a carrot, a cucumber and a banana all have in common? Give up? They are all, somehow, related to your passion, potency, or prostate. By now you know all about the carrots.

Cucumbers were once considered an aphrodisiac. The ancients believed in the doctrine of signatures, that is, the therapeutic efficacy of resemblances, and so anything with a phallic shape was assumed to assure potency.

Were you aware that certain situations could bring about impotence? Drinking can. You have a little and you feel like getting it on. You have a little more and you can't even get it up! For the social drinker who has too much, alcohol can be a temporary "downer." For the alcoholic, as mentioned previously, alcohol can permanently disrupt sexuality.

Certain high blood pressure medications lower more than your blood pressure! Impotence is supposedly not that common in males on blood pressure medication, but it does happen to some. (It probably happens to more. My guess is that a lot of "real men" wouldn't bring the subject up!) A lot of physicians don't discuss the potential side effects on potency for fear that bringing up the topic would drive "things" down. Well, that may be true. But what happens if you're one of the ones it happens to? You have no idea why you can't get it up. Just what a hypertensive man needs: one more thing to stress you out! Talk about a "downer!"

If you find yourself in this situation, don't stop taking your medication. Rather, discuss it with your physician, who'll most likely be able to work out another effective regimen for you. A change in dose or a switch to another drug is all you might need, but don't fool around with your medication without letting your doctor know. Keep in mind that untreated high blood pressure is called "the silent killer." Your primary goal is to avert a stroke, kidney failure or a heart attack. When you have your blood pressure under control, you can then deal with the other ups and downs.

What's considered high blood pressure? Here are some numbers for you:

Normal: 120/80 or less
Borderline: 140/90—160/95
High: Over 160/95

If yours is up, do something to get it down.

One "down" you need to deal with—if it's up—is your weight. For many people, dropping excess weight means a subsequent fall in blood pressure as well, which is why prevention-minded physicians usually suggest losing your lard. When you decide to trim down, you need to work with your physician so that your medication can be adjusted appropriately. Oftentimes, when you get your weight down to a reasonable level, you can get off your medication, and something else can get up! (Heh, Heh!) As we have seen, you don't even have to go on a diet to shed pounds—just cut down on fats and increase your fiber intake. (See "Strip and Undress," Chapter 20; "Fiber for Fluffies," Chapter 19; and "Take It Off," Chapter 21.)

Modern changes in our food supply have brought about a nasty nutritional shift that sets quite a few people up for blood pressure problems. When food is processed, salt (sodium chloride) goes in and potassium goes out, which unbalances the natural order of things. The contribution of excessive sodium and too little potassium can bring on high blood pressure problems in susceptible people.

A diet of fresh, minimally-processed foods provides you with all the sodium your body requires. (The exception might be in the compulsive type of individual who runs marathons in hot climates and steers clear of anything tainted with salt. That kind of person might not get enough to meet his/her needs!) The average American, however, is easily getting 10-20, even 30 times as much.

Shaking salt liberally on food is the obvious way to make salt intake go up. Reliance on convenience foods probably accounts for another giant share. Sodium lurks in things other than salt. It's in monosodium glutamate (marketed as Accent), sodium nitrate, sodium bicarbonate, sodium-whatever, and so on. So check out labels on packaged foods before you buy. (In the meantime, check out Table 22-1 to see which foods are the saltiest.)

Did you find any surprises on the list? One I find interesting is salad dressings. One tablespoon of the stuff can have as much as 150-300 mg of sodium, yet most people don't stop at a tablespoon... at least not at a salad bar! Two ladles (which adds up to 8 tablespoons) is more like it. But that means 1,200-2,400 mg a shot! That's a lot, considering that an ideal day's intake should be in the 2,500-3,500 mg range, and certainly below 5,000 mg! If you want a dressing that's completely salt free, you'll have to ask for oil and vinegar, straight up. Oil and vinegar-based dressings, such as Italian and the "house specials," are really loaded. But dressings are so high in fat content that it's best to reduce the amount you use anyway.

Another salt mine is fast food. Get this: A Big Mac contains 963 mg of sodium; a Quarterpounder with cheese has 1,206 mg. Are you

Table 22-1: Salty Selections

Add-to-Foods
- Salt, sea salt
- Seasoned salts (garlic salt, etc.)
- Accent, MSG
- Meat sauces
- Meat tenderizers
- Soy sauce
- Salad dressings

Convenience Foods
- Canned soups, vegetables and sauces
- Packaged dinners
- Vegetable juices
- Cake mixes

Deli Foods
- Luncheon meats, ham
- Sausage, bacon, corned beef
- Canned meats and fish
- Salted meats and fish
- Pickles, sauerkraut
- Processed cheeses and spreads
- Condiments

Fast Foods
- Burgers, hotdogs
- Fries
- Fried chicken
- Pizza

Instant Foods
- Dehydrated soups, bouillon cubes
- Instant cereals
- Instant sauces and dressings

Snack Foods
- Potato chips, pretzels
- Olives, jerkey
- Salted nuts, seeds
- Salted popcorn
- Salted crackers

ready for this one? At Dairy Queen the Super Brazier Hamburger packs a whopping 1,624 mg!

Cutting down doesn't mean you have to cut salt out completely. By emphasizing fresh foods and avoiding heavily processed foods, you'll automatically bring your salt intake in line. When cooking, add less than half the amount of salt the recipe calls for rather than putting it all in. If your recipe calls for a bouillon cube, then forget adding any additional salt. You can also use salt-free bouillon instead. Season your foods with herbs and spices, wine, garlic and onions. Take the salt shaker off the table. If you are a compulsive shaker, plug up the holes on your shaker!

If you think giving up salt is a bland affair, you're in for a real treat. You'll be better able to pick up the subtleties of flavor in foods. At first your taste buds might go into withdrawal—but take heart! The salty taste is an acquired one. After laying off the stuff for a while, you'll actually prefer foods that are less salty. It's fashionable now to shake salt habits, and marketing trends are following suit. A whole new line of reduced-sodium and salt-free products are coming on the market. Look for them when you shop.

Just as it's fairly easy to cut down on sodium, it's simple to boost your potassium intake. The best sources of potassium include:

- All fruits, not just oranges and bananas!
- Fresh and frozen vegetables provided there's no sauce or added salt
- Whole grains and pasta especially if you don't add salt to the cooking water
- Legumes (dried beans, peas and lentils)
- Unsalted nuts and seeds

These foods are the major ingredients of vegetarian fare and just for your information, a vegetarian diet has been found helpful in reducing blood pressure! So has a low fat diet, for that matter.

We've talked about carrots and cukes. What about the banana? It's high in potassium.

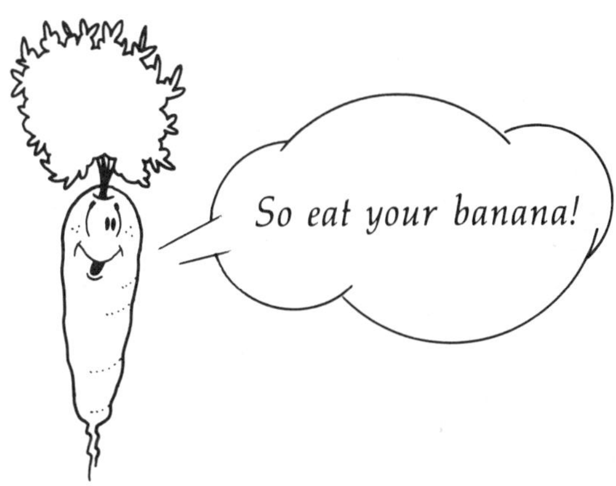

By the way, some recent research indicates that an inadequate calcium intake contributes to high blood pressure as well. So make sure you're getting enough. Check out Chapter 14, Breaking Up.

While we are talking about life's ups and downs, heed this. French researchers have reported in The Lancet, a British medical journal, that impotence may, in part, be related to high blood levels of cholesterol (over 280 mg/dl) and triglycerides (over 140 mg/dl). So don't let your diet break your heart or ruin your heartfelt expressions of love.

23

FLUID RELATIONSHIPS

No matter what you might think, it's not a good idea to avoid the wet spot! But unfortunately quite a few people do. I am not referring to one of "those" wet spots, but to the need to adequately replenish your body with fluids, particularly water. Water is, after all, more vital than food. We can go only two or three days without it.

Most people are just tall (short) drinks of water. If you're a woman, water constitutes 55-65% of your body weight. For men, it's higher: 65-75%. That's because men have more muscle mass. People with more muscle tissue contain more water, since a fluid environment is essential for optimal muscle function. Smart athletes understand that a lack of water impairs their performance. Even on an everyday basis, an inadequate water supply can lead to fatigue—and fatigue is not a boon to your sex life.

Your body altogether contains 40-50 quarts of water. During any given day, however, your body processes 10,000 quarts of water. Naturally most of it is recycled over and over again, but under ordinary circumstances you lose 2½-3 quarts daily. That's all you need to replace, but do you? You probably don't drink 12 cups of water a day. That's OK, because you don't have to. You'll get some water from your solid foods, because like you, they contain a lot of it. However, you will need to drink about 6-8 8-oz glasses of some fluid every day. Not all of that needs to be water, but I think most of it ought to be. After all, it has a big job to do. You need water for cooling, digestion, elimination and for preventing constipation. It "lubes" your joints and cushions your tissues.

With the variety of beverages available to us today, it's easy to forget H_2O. Drinks are sugarized, spirited, caffeinated, decaffeinated, herbed, mineralized and carbonated, but too much of any one type might be a problem. Too much soda and you get too much sugar or artificial sweetners. Too much booze and you're drunk. Too much caffeine and your nerves are on end. Too much decaf and you have to worry about the carcinogenicity of the solvent used in the decaffeinating process. Too much of the herbal stuff can lead to a variety of problems (see Table 23-1.) Mineralized and carbonated beverages can be a secret source of salt. However, the *only* time too much water is a problem is when your water supply is contaminated with disease-causing microorganisms or toxic contaminants. When water's pure, it's hard to get too much. The least you can do is drink four glasses of *water* daily, in addition to four of some other fluid! Just make sure your liquid libations consist of something besides java, sweetened drinks and hootch. Alcohol and caffeine exert a diuretic effect. Sugar increases your body's need for water.

If you're not thirsty for 8 cups/day, you need to know that thirst is only a fairly reliable indicator of your need for fluid. A study on athletes

Table 23—1: Herbal Perterbals

Herbal teas are enjoying a surge in popularity. Not all herbs are innocuous. Some may have negative effects because they contain powerful chemicals that can alter the functions of your body and mind. In fact, many modern drugs are derived from herbs and other plants. Since they are classified neither as foods nor drugs, herbs fall into a "gray area" and, as such, are not as well regulated as edibles and medications. In certain cultures the effects of herbs are well understood and respected. The average American does not have this wisdom and may get into trouble when using them.

ADVERSE PROPERTIES	HERBS
Allergenic	Chamomile, Goldenrod, Yarrow (if you're sensitive to ragweed, etc.) St. John's Wort
Carcinogens	Sassafras (Note: ordinary black tea contains tannin, a carcinogen linked to cancer of the esophagus and stomach. Adding milk to the tea inactivates tannin's carcinogenic effect.)
Cathartic	Senna, Buckthorn, Dock Roots, Aloe leaves
Diuretic	Buchu, Quackgrass, Dandelion (Note; their effect is not considered worse than that of coffee.)
Poisons	Indian Tobacco, Shave Grass (horsetail), Misletoe leaves
Toxins to the Nervous System	Catnip, Juniper, Hydrangea; Jimson Weed, Lobelia, Nutmeg, Wormwood

When packaged for use as tea, the concentration of active ingredients is fairly low and should pose little problem for the average healthy individual. The possibility of a hazardous reaction to an herbal tea preparation heightens when herbs are sold by the bulk. The potency of the tea depends upon several factors, including the part of the plant being used (leaf, stem or root), the strength of the brew and quantity and frequency of ingestion.

highlights the need to drink a little beyond your thirst: In an experiment at Harvard University, a group of athletes had to work out on a treadmill in a heated room. They got no water. Walking at a rate of 3 1/2 miles/hour, they became exhausted in 3½ hours. A few days later, they repeated the exercise, except that this time they were allowed to drink as much as they felt they needed. There was a dramatic improvement in performance. This time they went six hours before they tuckered out. Then, when they were forced to drink the same amount of water as their bodies actually lost, guess what happened: They kept going for another hour! If you're chronically fatigued, you might be slightly, albeit chronically, dehydrated.

Excessive consumption of caffeinated beverages (see Table in "Breast Bumps," Chapter 11) can cause a variety of troubles from heartburn to fast heartbeats and abnormal heart rhythms. You've seen people with coffee nerves. Ten to twenty cups of a strong coffee a day can cause symptoms that are easily mistaken for an anxiety attack. People strung out on coffee don't exactly look like they're ready to relax in bed, etc. There is even some concern that excessive coffee consumption by pregnant women can cause fetal abnormalities. Some preliminary studies have linked heavy-duty coffee-cupping to an increased risk of miscarriage, stillbirth and premature birth. In addition to all this, caffeine jeopardizes your B-vitamin status, masks fatigue and contributes to low blood sugar problems. Wouldn't you agree that one to two cups is truly enough? If you're a frequent worshipper at the sacred coffee urn at work, why not head off to the drinking fountain instead?

The subject of alcohol has come up several times already. In large amounts, it does nothing for your sex life—except ruin it. Pregnant women who drink heavily give birth to children with an array of abnormalities (including physical deformities and mental retardation), which has subsequently been dubbed "fetal alcohol syndrome." Because of that, physicians advise pregnant women to avoid alcohol, or to at least restrict it to two drinks a day or less.

If you're not alcoholic, a drink in a pleasant atmosphere with a lover or friends is a very pleasurable experience. Don't push drinks on others, though. They know what's best for themselves. There are a lot more people with alcohol-related difficulties than you would think, and most of them are regular people, just like you and me. If you're giving a party, make sure a variety of non-alcoholic beverages are readily available for friends who prefer not to drink. Don't let yourself be bamboozled into drinking when you don't want to, either. And by all means, avoid guzzling the stuff down too quickly.

Your liver needs about an hour to process the alcohol in a typical drink (a 12-oz beer, 4 oz of wine, a 1½-oz jigger of 80 proof spirits). If you're downing drinks at a faster rate than your liver can process the stuff, alcohol builds up in your bloodstream. First you feel high and carefree. Then you get clumsy and drunk. If you get in your car, you're a hazard. If you make it home, you might not be any good in bed! Coffee and a cold shower won't sober you up—only time will. Even so, when the morning rolls around you might find yourself saying

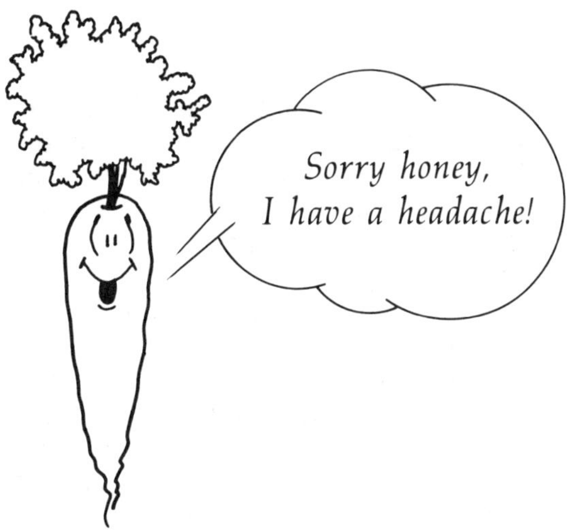

24

VARY YOUR POSITIONS

Eating, like sex, gets a little boring if you seldom change the menu. After all, variety is the spice of life, and no matter what it is you're doing, getting in a rut closes off a lot of living. When it comes to keeping yourself well nourished, the same is true. The more limited your diet, the more you miss out on the esthetic, sensual and nutritional value of wholesome foods.

You could go to the store and purchase hundreds of food products, yet bring a very limited amount of basic foods into your home. Most of the products available on market shelves today are composites of three major ingredients: sugar, white flour and fat. That goes for cookies, crackers, cakes, cake mixes, packaged pancake mix, biscuits, cereals and even some dietetic meal replacements. They come in an array of sizes, shapes and colors. The most impressive part about them is the detail in the packaging. If you have a question about the nutritional value of a new food product, here are two guidelines to follow:

> *Number One:* The better the package, the worse the nutritional value!
> *Number Two:* Never eat anything that glows in the dark! "Real foods" aren't phosphorescent.

These rules may at times be more reliable than reading the label. Many of the flour-fat-sugar combos have a bunch of vitamins added back to "fortify" them. Most of the time there's no need to fortify anything that's not weakened in the first place. (The exception here is fortified milk, which is wholesome.) Just think about the chippy-whippys, the flakos, etc. Would you be proud to offer them to George Washington if he were around here today? Can you see yourself saying, "Mr. President, care for a Ding-Dong?" Vitamins added to this kind of product cannot make up for the fact that it's still a highly processed refined food. *Au contraire,* take an orange or a broccoli. They speak for themselves. You know they have integrity. Basic food has been around for eons. You can't say the same for factory foods that bear little nutritional resemblance to the foods from which they were derived.

While shopping, vary your position in the store by developing "off the wall" shopping habits. Most markets have the fresh foods on the outer walls and the processed foods stacked up in the interior aisles. Spend most of your time going around the outside. Occasionally go down an aisle to pick up some staples: beans, oatmeal and, of course, toilet paper since you're into fiber now. You'll spend less time in the store—after all, you won't have to make any earthshaking decisions as to whether you want your chips ruffled, or as stackable disks. In today's world it helps to simplify things whenever you can. Getting back to basics with food is no exception. The payoff is less time in the store and most likely more time added to your life! You'll just be a whole lot healthier if you eat a variety of whole grains, vegetables, fruits and low-fat, protein-containing foods (legumes, lean meats, poultry, fish and dairy products.)

The next time you eat, look at your plate. What relative positions do the high fat and high fiber foods take?

Breakfast:

If yours is fried eggs, buttered white bread and juice, you have a few alternatives.

If you want to keep it similar, have poached eggs on unbuttered whole-grain toast and a piece of fruit. The fat went from a hefty 35 grams to 10. Fiber shot up from less than 2 grams to almost 5.

If you're interested in a big fiber boost, do this instead: Have some fruit, a dish of cereal with some milk and a bran muffin. Depending on your choice of cereal and fruit, you can get almost ten times as much fiber in the A.M. (And that will pay off later in a BM!)

Breakfast—Skipper's Special:

If you hate eating first thing in the morning and wait till you get to work for your doughnut or sweet roll, here's a suggestion for you: How about brown-bagging a banana along with a small peanut butter sandwich on whole wheat or a bran muffin. Not only will you fiber up, you'll also avoid ups and downs in your blood sugar brought about by an infusion of sugar and caffeine.

Lunch:

If you tend to go for burgers and sandwiches, usually you'll encounter bread or a bun or bagel with a huge hunk of dark meat inside along with a millimeter of tomato and a lot of mayo. That, too, can give you a low fiber reading (less than 2 grams) and a large lard load logging in 50 grams of fat!

Do this instead: Take heavy-duty whole-grain bread and fill

it with two ounces of white meat (poultry, tuna) or even a garbanzo spread (hummus). Add some thick tomato slices, deep green lettuce, some sprouts and a tad of mayo. Your fat's below 10 grams, and fiber's over 6. Toss in a carrot and an apple for a little crunch and you add another 6 grams of fiber! Buy a carton of skim or lowfat milk for a beverage.

Dinner:

Are you the kind that has a huge piece of meat that's so big it takes up more than half your dinner plate?

Your meat (fish, poultry) portion should fit into a wedge that's only a quarter or even an eighth of your plate. Admittedly, it does look lonely out there. So add some hefty portions of grains or spuds (1 cup), and another 2 cups of vegetables. Add a salad and a dish of fruit. That brings your fiber close to 20 grams. Meanwhile your fat has toppled from a whopping 80-100 grams (for a 10-oz. hunk of well-marbled beef) to less than 20!

This gives you a fiber intake that's compatible with a reduced risk of both heart disease and cancer. One way to keep your sex life alive is to keep yourself alive . . . and well! As you've already seen, these foods are vital for prostates, vaginas, breasts, testicles, sperms, eggs—whatever you've got!

The wonderful aspect of varying your positions is that you are enriched by the process, not deprived. There's more color, more crunch, more texture and more nutrients. There's less fat, more fiber and a whole lot more to chew. Eating these kinds of foods satisfies "mouth hunger" by giving your teeth something to sink into. Yummm.

Does this mean you can never have an ice cream or a piece of cheesecake? Good heavens, no. One position you need to get off is the one marked "do it all or do nothing." This is when you decide that from Monday on, you will always eat the "good" stuff and never touch the "bad" stuff ever, ever again. As soon as you have a bite of something you think is "bad," you forget the whole thing. Doing it all, 100% of the time, does not work for most mortals. In fact it's often counterproductive, because you'll wind up doing nothing.

When you give yourself a little leeway, dietary changes are not as threatening. Have a scoop of ice cream during the week. That certainly beats a gallon every day. Put it in perspective. A bit of rich food every now and then is not a problem when your overall eating pattern is low in fat and high in fiber. If you eat foods that are consistent with good health and weight control 75-85% of the time, you'll feel healthier and be more energetic. There's a big difference between "daily bread" and a "treat." When your treats are truly treats, and not everyday fare, you'll appreciate them even more. Incidentally, make those treats worthy of you. Don't settle for junk. Select something special, delicious and expensive. Why settle for less? It's better to have the best infrequently than a steady diet of mediocrity.

One last thing: Take the judgmental labels off food. Foods are neither good nor bad. For most people "good" means "carte blanche"—i.e., "Eat as much as you want." After all, "It's good for you!" Wrong! Case in point: Take safflower oil. It's health-promoting when eaten in tiny amounts. Fry everything you eat in it, and you have a diet that's very high in fat. Up goes your risk for breast or prostate cancer, not to mention that you'd be a likelier target for a heart attack.

The "bad" list of forbidden foods makes you eat more in the long run. When you eat a "bad" food, you transfer the moral judgement to yourself. That makes you a "bad" person. Now you feel guilty, so what do you do? Eat more! Oy vay! Some foods are junky, nutritionally-depleted, and loaded with calories. Call them what they are, don't call them "bad." When you "calls them as you sees them," it just might be easier to avoid a few.

Here's an idea that's neither good nor bad, just smart. Keep your evening meal light. If you eat a very heavy dinner, chances are you won't feel sexy at bedtime. It's hard to float heavenly in the arms of your lover when you're praying for a hole in the mattress in which you can drop your loaded stomach.

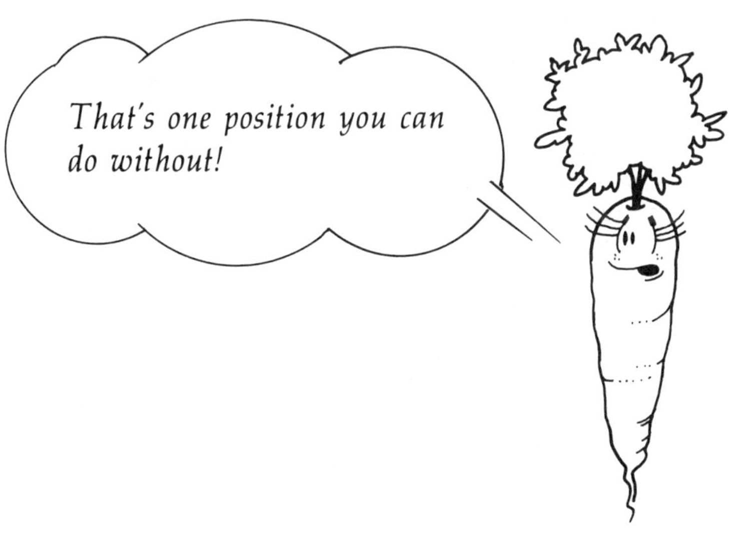

25

PROPHYLACTIC MASTICATIONS

Sounds dirty, doesn't it? It's something worth doing frequently, however. "Prophylactic," of course, is an adjective. It means "preventive." (That's why "those" things got "that" name.) "Prophylactic" modifies the noun "mastication," which means "chewing." Prophylactic mastication is a preventive health habit concerning what you "chews" in life.

Food is glorious. Look at the variety in color, form, aroma, texture and taste. Imagine the almost limitless scrumptious combinations. Be thankful for all the edible beauty that nourishes you and keeps you well. Respect it. Keep it whole. A lot of people don't.

Hundreds of food products are made from foods that have been highly refined. Little of their original nutritional value is left for you. There's some effort to restore what's lost, but it's never enough. At best we can only restore what we know is lost, and most of the time we don't even do that much. Nutrition as a science is relatively new; food is eons older by comparison. We have not even come close to understanding the incredible complexity of the simple foods we eat.

Proteins, vitamins and minerals are just the beginning of the story, not the end. There's fiber, recently rediscovered. It's always been there for us; we just didn't appreciate its importance, because it wasn't like the other nutrients. We assumed that if we couldn't pin down its function, it had none. In addition to fiber, several other "new" food components have been discovered: indoles, protease inhibitors, chlorophyll—all of which have anti-cancer properties. Are there other healthful food factors? Most likely! How can you get them? Eat and enjoy real, wholesome foods.

While supplementary nutrients are highly beneficial at times, bottled nutrients cannot replace basic food. We will probably never be able to fabricate anything as wonderful as a green pepper or a bing cherry. I think that's because our products are mere fabrications, not divine creations. Somehow, overly refined food and nutrient-pills are missing the very essence of life itself, the soul.

That's why real food has got to be the center of your nutritional experience.

No matter how divine food is, eating is still an earthy thing to do. I suggest you prophylactically masticate something several times a day.

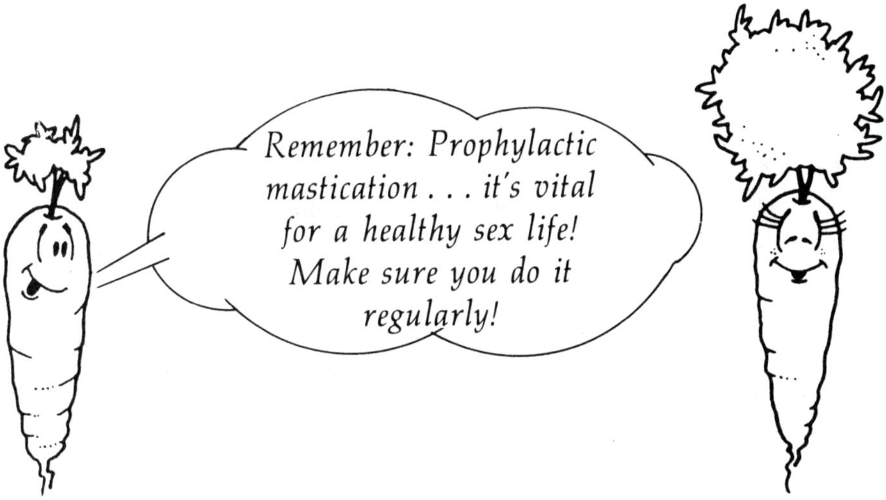
Remember: Prophylactic mastication . . . it's vital for a healthy sex life! Make sure you do it regularly!

RESOURCES

ALCOHOLISM

Marshall, J.A. *Find Your Perfect High.* Glendale, CA: Happy Eye Enterprises, 1978.

EXERCISE/SEX

White, James, R. *Exercise and Sexual Response in Men.* (In press: write to author at UCSD, Department of Physical Education, La Jolla, CA 92037 for more information.)

HERPES

Herpes Research Club
The Saturday Evening Post Society
1100 Waterbury Road
Indianapolis, Indiana 46202

MAGAZINES & NEWSLETTERS

American Health Magazine (80 Fifth Avenue, New York, NY 10011)
Medical Self Care (P.O. Box 717, Inverness, CA 94937)
Nutrition Action (CSPI, 1755 S St., NW, Washington, D.C. 20009)

NUTRITION

General:

Brody, Jane. *Jane Brody's Nutrition Book.* New York: Norton, 1981.
Cumming, Candy; Newman, Vicky. *Eater's Guide: Nutrition Basics for Busy People.* Englewood Cliffs, NJ: Prentice-Hall, 1981.

Vegetarian:

Robertson, Laurel; Flinders, C.; Godfrey, Bronwen. *Laurel's Kitchen.* New York: Bantam Books (paperback), 1978; or Petaluma, CA: Nilgiri Press (hardcover), 1976.

For Sports:
Coleman, Ellen. *Eating for Endurance.* Riverside, CA: Rubidoux Co., 1980. Available from: California Dietetic Association, P.O. Box 3506, Santa Monica, CA 90403.

PREMENUSTRUAL TENSION SYNDROME (PMS)

Premenstrual Blues. Available from: Optimox, Inc., P.O. Box 3378, Torrance, CA 90510.

MENOPAUSE

"Midlife Wellness: A Journal for the Middle Years" from Center for Climacteric Studies, University of Florida, 901 N.W. 8th Avenue, Suite B-1, Gainesville, Florida 32601

WEIGHT CONTROL

Bailey, Covert. *Fit or Fat.* Boston: Houghton Mifflin Company, 1978.
Bennet, William; Gurin, Joel. *The Dieter's Dilemma.* New York: Basic Books, Inc., 1982.
Katahn, Martin. *The 200 Calorie Solution.* New York: Norton, 1982.

BIBLIOGRAPHY

Abraham, G. E. "Premenstrual Tension," *Current Problems in Obstetrics and Gynecology*, 1980, *3*, 1-39.

Abraham, C.; Lubran, M. "Serum and Red Cell Magnesium Levels in Patients with Premenstrual Tension." *American Journal of Clinical Nutrition, 1981, 34*, 2364-2366.

Abraham, G.; Schwartz, U.; Lubran, M. "Effect of Vitamin B-6 on Plasma and Red Blood Cell Magnesium Levels in Premenopausal Women." *Annals of Clinical and Laboratory Science*, 1981, *11*, 333-336.

Abraham, G. "The Premenstrual Tension Syndromes." *Contemporary Obstetric and Gynecological Nursing*, 1980, *111*, 170-184.

Abraham, G.; Hargrove, J. "Effect of Vitamin B-6 on Premenstrual Symptomalogy in Women with Premenstrual Tension Syndromes: a Double Blind Crossover Study." *Infertility*, 1980, *3*, 155-165.

Abraham, G. "Magnesium Deficiency in Premenstrual Tension." *Magnesium Bulletin*, 1982, *1*, 68-73.

Adams, P. M.; Rose, D. P.; Folkard, V., et al. "Effect of Pyridoxine Hydrochloride (Vitamin B-6) upon Depression Associated with Oral Contraception." *The Lancet*, 1973, April 28, 897.

Alderson, M. R. "Prostate Cancer—Epidemiology." *Recent Results in Cancer Research*, 1981, *78*, 1-15.

Amelar, R.; Dublin, L.; Schoenfeld, C. "Sperm Motility." *Fertility and Sterility*, 1980, *34*, 197-215.

Amelar, R. *Infertility in Men: Diagnosis and Treatment.* Philadelphia: F. A. Davis Company, 1966.

Anderson, James W. *Diabetes: a Practical New Guide to Healthy Living.* New York: Arco Publishing Company, 1981.

Anon. "Premenstrual Syndrome." *The Lancet*, 1981, December 19/26, 1393-1394.

Anon. "Progress on Pyridoxine." *Nutrition and the M.D.*, 1980, *6*, 4-5.

Anon. "Prolonged Use of the 'Pill' Linked to Skin Cancer." *San Diego Union.* May 17, 1983.

Anon. "The Vitamin B-6 Requirement in Oral Contraceptive Users." *Nutrition Reviews*, 1979, *37*, 344-345.

Anon. "Dysmenorrhea: Effective New Approach to a Controversial Problem." *Medical Journal of Australia,* 1980, March 22, 248-249.

Anon. "A gland for No Reason?" *The Harvard Medical School Health Letter.* 1980, March.

Anon. "Vitamin A, Tumor Initiation and Tumor Promotion." *Nutrition Reviews*, 1979, *37*, 153-156.

Anon. "High Protein Diets and Bone Homeostasis. *Nutrition Reviews,* 1981, *39*, 11-13.

Anon. "A pain in the head." *Harvard Medical School Health Letter*, 1979, December.

Anon. "Vitamin E for Hot Flashes." *Journal of the American Medical Association*, 1958, *167*, 1806.

Avioli, L. V. "Postmenopausal Osteoporosis: Prevention Versus Cure." *Federation Proceedings*, 1981, *40*, 2418-2422.

Bailey, Covert, *Fit or Fat.* Boston: Houghton Mifflin Company, 1978.

Bennett, William; Gurin, Joel. *The Dieter's Dilemma*. New York; Basic Books, Inc., 1982.

Barzel, U. S. "Osteoporosis in Young Men. *Archives of Internal Medicine*, 1982, *142*, 2079.

Basu, T. K. "Vitamin A and Cancer of Epithelial Origin." *Journal of Human Nutrition*, 1979, *33*, 24-31.

Berkow, R.; Talbott, J. H., eds. *The Merck Manual of Diagnosis and Treatment.* Rathway, NJ: Merck Sharp and Dohme Research laboratories, 1977.

Bermond, P. "Therapy of Side Effects of Oral Contraceptive Agents with Vitamin B-6." *Acta Vitaminologica Enzymologica*, 1982, *4*, 45-54..

Bieri, J. G.; Corash, L.; Hubbard, V. A. "Medical Uses of Vitamin E. New England Journal of Medicine, 1983, *308*, 1063-1072.

Bogart, J.; Briggs, G.; Calloway, D. *Nutrition and Physical Fitness.* Philadelphia: W. B. Saunders Company, 1973.

Bosse, T. R.; Donald, E. A. "The Vitamin B-6 Requirement in Oral Contraceptive Users." *American Journal of Clinical Nutrition*, 1979, *32*, 1015-1023.

Brainard, J. B. *Control of Migraine.* New York: W. W. Norton and Company, Inc., 1977.

Bray, G., ed. *Obesity in America.* Washington, DC USDHEW NIH publication no. 79-359, 1979.

Brody, J. *Jane Brody's Nutrition Book.* New York: W. W. Norton, 1981.

Brooks, P. G.; Gart, S.; Heldfond, A. J. "Measuring the Effect of

Caffeine Restriction in Fibrocystic Breast Disease." *Journal of Reproductive Medicine*, 1981, *26*, 279-282.

Brush, M. G. "Efamol in the Treatment of the Premenstrual Syndrome." 1981, unpublished.

Burkitt, Dennis. *Eat Right—to Stay Healthy and Enjoy Life More.* New York: Arco Publishing Company, 1979.

Bush, I. M., et al. Report to American Urological Association meeting, 1972 and to the American Medical Association meeting, 1974.

Caldamone, A. A.; Freytag, M. K.; Cockett, A. T. "Seminal Zinc and Male Infertility. *Urology*, 1979, *8*, 280-281.

Check, W. A., "Folate for Oral Contraceptive Users May Reduce Cervical Cancer Risk." *Journal of the American Medical Association*, 1980, *244*, 633-634.

Chopra, D. P.; Wilkoff, L. J. "Inhibition and Reversal by B-Retinoic Acid of Hyperplasia Induced in Cultured Mouse Prostate Tissues by 3-Methylcholanthrene or N-Methyl-N-Nitro-N-Nitrosoguanidine. *Journal of the National Cancer Institute*, 1976, *56*, 583-589.

Chow, C. K. "Nutritional Influence on Cellular Antioxidant Defense Systems." *American Journal of Clinical Nutrition*, 1979, *32*, 1066-1081.

Christy, C. "Vitamin E in Menopause.' *American Journal of Obstetrics and Gynecology*, 1945, *50*, 84-87.

Cogwill, U. M. "Selenium and Human Fertility. *"Proceedings of the Symposium on Selenium-Tellurium in the Environment*, 1976.

Cumming, C.; Newman, V. *Eater's Guide: Nutrition Basics for Busy People.* Englewood Cliffs, NJ: Prentice-Hall, Inc., 1981.

Dalton, K. *The Premenstrual Syndrome.* London: Heinemann, 1964.

DeCosse, J.: "Potential for Chemoprevention. *"Cancer*, 1982, *50*, 2250-2253 (Supplement).

deWaard, F. "Relationship of Weight to the Promotion of Breast Cancer After Menopause." *Nutrition and Cancer, 1982, 4*, 85-88.

Diezel, W.; Engel, S.; Sonnichsen, N.; Hohne, W. E., "Lipid Peroxidation Products in Human Spermatozoa: Detection and Pathogenic Significance." *Andrologia*, 1980, *12*, 167-171.

Dougherty, R. C.; Whitaker, M. J.; Smith, L. M., et al. "Negative Chemical Ionization Studies of Human and Food Chain Contamination with Xenobiotic Chemicals." *Environmental Health Perspectives*, 1980, *36*, 103-118.

Fair, W. R. "The Prostatic Antibacterial Factor: Identity and Significance." *Prostatic Diseases*, Marberger, H. et al., eds, New York: Alan R. Liss, Inc., 1976.

Fazio, V. "Acute Effects of Alcohol on Plasma Ascorbic Acid in Healthy Subjects." *American Journal of Clinical Nutrition*, 1981, *34*, 2394-2396.

Findlay, S.; Liebman, B. "Brittle Bones." *Nutrition Action*, 1982, *9*,

12-13.
Finkle, A. L. "What Dietary Restrictions for Benign Prostatic Hypertrophy?" *Journal of the American Medical Association*, 1976, *236*, 2669-2670.
Finkler, R. S. "The Effect of Vitamin E in the Menopause." *Journal of Clinical Endocrinology and Metabolism*, 1949, *9*, 89-94.
Frost, D.; Lish, P.M." Selenium in Biology." *Annual Review of Pharmacology*, 1975, *15*, 259-284.
Gantt, P. A.; McDonough, P. G. "Adolescent Dysmenorrhea." *The Pediatric Clinics of North America*, 1981, *28*, 389-395.
Gershoff, S. N., Prien, E. L. "Effect of Daily MgO and Vitamin B-6 Administration to Patients with Recurring Calcium Oxalate Kidney Stones." *American Journal of Clinical Nutrition*, 1967, 20, 393.
Goei, G.; Abraham, G. "Effect of a Nutritional Supplement, Optivite for Women, on Premenstrual Symptomology in Patients with Premenstrual Tension." *Journal of Reproductive Medicine*, 1983.
Goei, G.; Raltson, J.; Abraham, G. "Dietary Patterns of Patients with Premenstrual Tension," *Journal of Applied Nutrition*, 1982, *34*, 4-9.
Gonzalez, E. R. "Premenstrual Syndrome: an Ancient Woe Deserving of Modern Scrutiny." *Journal of the American Medical Association*, 1981, *245*, 1393-1396.
Goodhart, R., Shils, M. *Modern Nutrition in Health and Disease*. Philadelphia: Lea and Febiger, 1981.
Gordon, E. F., *Pediatrics*, 1981, *99*, 341-349.
Gordon, R. C.; Passal, D. B. "Zinc Metabolism: Basic Clinical and Behavioral Aspects."
Gozan, H. A. "The Use of Vitamin E in Treatment of the Menopause." *New York State Journal of Medicine*, 1952, *52*, 1289-1291.
Griffith, R. S.; Norins, A. L.; Kagan, C. "A Multicentered Study of Lysine Therapy in Herpes Simplex Infection." *Dermatologica*, 1978, *156*, 257-267.
Guthrie, B. E. "Chromium, Manganese, Copper, Zinc, Cadmium Content of New Zealand Foods." *New Zealand Medical Journal*, 1975, 418-424.
Habib, F. K.; Hammond, G. L.; Lee, I. R., et al. "Metal-Androgen Interrelationships in Carcinoma and Hyperplasia of the Human Prostate." *Journal of Endocrinology*, 1976, *71*, 133-14.
Hambridge, K. M.; Hambridge, C.; Jacobs, M.; Baum, J. D. "Low Levels of Zinc in Hair, Anorexia, Poor Growth and Hypogeusia in Children." *Pediatrics Research*, 1972, *6*, 868.
Hargrove, J.; Abraham, G. "Effects of Vitamin B-6 on Infertility in Women with the Premenstrual Tension Syndrom." *Infertility*, 1979, *2*, 315-322.
Harris, W. A.; Harden, T. E.; Dawson, E. B. "Apparent Effect of Ascorbic Acid Medication on Semen Metal Levels." *Fertility and Sterility*, 1979, *32*, 455-450.

Hartoma, T. R.; Nahoul, K.; Netter, A., "Zinc, Plasma Androgens and Male Sterility." *The Lancet*, 1977, November 26, 1125-1126.

Hicks, M. "The Scientific Basis for Regarding Vitamin A and Its Analogues as Anti-Carcinogenic Agents." *Proceedings of the Nutrition Society*, 1983, *42*, 83-93.

Hill, P.; Wydner, E. L.; Garnes, H.; Walker, A. R. P. "Environmental Factors, Hormone Status and Prostate Cancer." *Preventive Medicine*, 1980, *9*, 657-666.

Hill, P.; Garbaczewski, L.; Helman, P. "Diet, Lifestyle and Menstrual Activity." *American Journal of Clinical Nutrition*, 1980, *33*, 1192-1198.

Hinton, M. A., et al. "Eating Behavior and Dietary Intake of Girls 2-14 Years Old. Psychologic, Sociologic and Physiologic Factors." *Journal of American Diet Association*, 1965, *43*, 223.

Hiryama, T. "Epidemiology of Prostate Cancer with Special Reference to the Role of Diet." *National Cancer Institute Monograph*, #53, 1979, 149-155.

Hodges, R. E., ed. *Nutrition: Metabolic and Clinical Applications.* New York: Plenum Press, 1979.

Holden, J.; Wolf, W.; Mertz, W. "Zinc and Copper in Self-Selected Diets." *Journal of the American Dietetic Association*, 1979, *75*, 23-28.

Hogan, B. "Epithelial Cancer, Differentiation, and Vitamin A." *Nature*, 1979, *277*, 261-262.

Hudiburgh, N. K.; Milner, A. N. "Influence of Oral Contraceptives on Ascorbic Acid and Triglyceride Status." *American Journal of Clinical Nutrition, 1979, 75*, 19-22.

Johansson, G., "Magnesium and Renal Stone Disease." *Acta Medica Scandinavica* (Supplement), 1982, *661* 13-18.

Kane, F. J. Evaluation of Emotional Reactions to Oral Contraceptives." *American Journal of Obstetrics and Gynecology*, 1976, *126*, 968-72.

Katahn, Martin. *The 200 Calorie Solution*. New York: Norton, 1982.

Kavinoky, N. R. "Vitamin E and the Control of Climacteric Symptoms." *Annals of Western Medicine and Surgery*, 1950, *4*, 27-32.

Kenmann, E.; Pasquale, S.; Skaf, R. "Amenorrhea Associated with Carotenemia." *Journal of the American Medical Association*, 1983, *249*, 926-929.

Klevay, L.; Peck S., Barcomme, D. "Evidence of Copper and Zinc Deficiency." *Journal of the American Medical Association*, 1979, *241*, 1916-1918.

Kromhout, D.; Bosschieter, E.; de Lezenne Coulander, C. "Dietary Fiber and 10-year Mortality from Coronary Heart Disease, Cancer and All Causes." *The Lancet*, 1982, September 4, 518-521.

Kummerow, F. A. "Nutrition Imbalance and Angiotoxins as Dietary Risk Factors in Coronary Heart Disease. *American Journal Clinical*

Nutrition, 1979, *32*, 58-83.

Lamano Carvalho, T. L.; Lopes, R. A.; Azoubel, R. "Morphometric Study of Testicle Alterations in Rats Submitted to Hypervitaminosis." *International Journal for Vitamin and Nutrition Research*, 1978, *48,* 307-315.

Lamano, Carvalho, T. L.; Lopes, R. A.; Azoubel, R. "Morphometric Study of the Reversibility of Testicle Alterations in Rats Submitted to Hypervitaminosis A." *International Journal for Vitamin and Nutrition Research*, 1978, *48*, 316-324.

Lemann, J.; Adams, N.; Gray, R. N. "Urinary Calcium Excretion in Human Beings." *New Englandd Journal of Medicine*, 1979, *301*, 535.

Levander, O. "Selenium and Chromium in Human Nutrition. *Journal of the American Diet Association*, 1975, *66*, 338-344.

Lindenbaum, J.; Whitehead, N.; Reyner, F. "Oral Contraceptive Hormones, Folate Metabolism, and the Cervical Epithelium." *American Journal of Clinical Nutrition*, 1975, *28*, 345-353.

London, R. S.; Sundaram, G. S.; Schultz, M., et al. "Endocrine Parameters and Alpha Tocopherol Therapy of Patients with Mammary Dysplasia." *Cancer Research*, 1981, *41*, 3811-3813.

Lopez, R. "Riboflavin Deficiency in an Adolescent Population in New York City. *American Journal of Clinical Nutrition*, 1980, *33*, 1283-1286.

Lopez, R. et al. "Riboflavin Deficiency in a Pediatric Population of Low Socioeconomic Status in New York City. *Journal of Pediatrics*, 1975, *87*, 420.

Love, S. M.; Gelman, R. S.; Silen, W. "Fibrocystic 'Disease' of the Breast: a Nondisease?" *New England JOurnal of Medicine*, 1982, *307*, 1010-1014.

Lucis, O. J.; Aterman, K. "Tumorigenesis by Cadmium." *Oncology* 1972, *26*, 53-67.

Mahajan, S. K. "Effect of Oral Zinc Therapy on Gonadal Function in Hemodialysis Patients." *Annals of Internal Medicine*, 1982, *97* 357-361.

March, D. C. *Handbook: Interactions of Selected Drugs and Nutritional Status in Man.* Chicago: The American Dietetic Assoc., 1976.

Marmar, J. L.; Katz, S.; Praiss, D. E. "Semen Zinc Levels in Infertile and Postvasectomy Patients and Patients with Prostatitis." *Fertility and Sterility*, 1975, *26*, 1057-1062.

Marsh, A. G.; Sanchez, T. V.; Chaffee, F. L., et al. "Bone Mineral Mass in Adult Lacto-Ovo Vegetarian and Omniverous Males." *American Journal of Clinical Nutrition*, 1983, *37*, 453-456.

Massey, L. K.; Davison, M. A. "Effects of Oral Contraceptives on Nutritional Status." *American Family Physician*, 1979, *19*, 119.

McConnell, K. P.; Burton, R. M., "Selenium and spermatogenesis." *Selenium in Biology and Medicine*, 1981.

Milman, N.; Scheibel, J.; Jessen, O. "Lysine Prophylaxis in Recurrent Herpes Simplex Labialis: a Double-Blind, Controlled Crossover Study." *Acta Dermato-Venereologica*, 1980, *60*, 85-87.

Minton, J. P.; Foecking, M. K.; Webster, D. J. T., et al. "Caffeine, Cyclic Nucleotides and Breast Disease." *Surgery*, 1979, *86*, 105-109.

Minton, J. P.; Abou-Issa, H.; Reiches, N.; Roseman, J. M. "Clinical and Biochemical Studies on Methyixanthine-related Fibrocystic Breast Disease." *Surgery*, 1981, *90*, 299-304.

Moghissi, K. S.; Evans, T. N. *Nutritional Impacts on Women*, New York: Harper and Row, 1977.

Murthy, N. K.; Vijaya, S. "Vitamin Nutritional Status of Women Using Oral Contraceptive Pills." *Indian Journal of Nutrition and Dietetics*, 1980, *17*, 79.

Newell, G. R.; Ellison, N. M., eds. *Nutrition and Cancer: Etiology and Treatment*. New York: Raven Press, 1981.

Newman, L. J. "Riboflavin Deficiency in Women Taking Oral Contraceptive Agents." *American Journal of Clinical Nutrition*, 1978, *31*, 247.

Ovesen, L. "Drugs and Vitamin Deficiency." *Drugs*, 1979, *18*, 278-298.

Owen, W. L. "Cancer of the Prostate: a Literature Review." *Journal of Diseases*, 1976, *29*, 89-114.

Piscator, M. "Role of Cadmium in Carcinogenesis with Special References to Cancer of the Prostate." *Environmental Health Perspectives*, 1981, *40*, 107-120.

Piterman, L.; Marks, R. "Herpes Simplex Infections: a Combined GP and Specialist View. *Australian Family Physician*, 1982, *11*, 197-202.

Pitts, G. C. "Factors Affecting Work Output in Hot Environment." *American Journal of Physiology* 1944, *142*, 254.

Puska, P., et al. "Controlled Randomized Trial of the Effect of Dietary Fat on Blood Pressure." *Lancet*, 1983, January 8, 1-5.

Reddy, B. S.; Cohen, L. A..; McCoy, G. D., et al. "Nutrition and Its Relationship to Cancer." *Advances in Cancer Research*, 1980, *32*, 282-329.

Reid, R. L.; Yen, S. C. "Premenstrual Syndrome." *American Journal of Obstetrics and Gynecology*, 1981, *139*, 85-104.

Roe, D. "Drug-induced Deficiency of B Vitamins." *New York State Journal of Medicine*, 1971, *27*, 702-776.

Romney, S. L.; Palen, P. R.; Duttagupta, C. "Retinoids and the Prevention of Cervical Dysplasia." *American Journal of Obstetrics and Gynecology*, 1981, *141*, 890-894.

Rouse, I., et. al. "Blood Pressure Lowering Effect of a Vegetarian Diet: Controlled Trial in Normotensive Subjects." *The Lancet*, 1983, January 8, 5-10.

Russell, R. M.; Boyer, J. L. "Hepatic Injury from Chronic Hypervitaminosis A Resulting in Portal Hypertension and Acidosis." *New England Journal of Medicine*, 1974, *291*, 435.

Sanstead, H. "Zinc Nutrition in the United States." *American Journal of Clinical Nutrition*, 1973, *26*, 1251-1260.

Saturday Evening Post Society. *Keeping Posted on Herpes.* Indianapolis: The Benjamin Franklin Literary and Medical Society, series 1, no. 1.

Schroeder, H. "Losses of Vitamins and Trace Minerals Resulting from Processing and Preservation of Foods." *American Journal of Clinical Nutrition*, 1971, *24*, 562-73.

Schauzer, G. N.; White, D. A.; Schneider, C. J., "Cancer Mortality Correlation Studies, III: Statistical Associations with Dietary Selenium Intakes." *Bioinorganic Chemistry*, 1977, *7*, 23-31.

Seelig, M. S. "Magnesium Requirements in Human Nutrition." *Contemporary Nutrition*, 1982, 7, 1-2.

Seelig, M. S. *Magnesium Deficiency in the Pathogenesis of Disease.* New York: Plenum Medical Books Company, 1980.

Shamberger, R. "Antioxidants and Cancer." *Archives of Ennvironmental Health*, 1976, *31*, 231-235.

Skandhan, K. P.; Skandhan, S.; Mehta, Y. B. "Semen Electrolytes in Normal and Infertile Subjects. II. Zinc." *Experientia*, 1978, *34*, 1476-1478.

Solomons, N. W. "Factors Affecting the Bioavailability of Zinc." *Journal of the American Dietetic Association*, 1982, *80*, 115-121.

Stange, L.; Carlstrom, K.; Eriksson, M. "Hypervitaminosis A in Early Human Pregnancy and Malformations of the Central Nervous System." *Acta Obstetrica et Gynecologica Scandinavica*, 1978, *57*, 289-91.

Sundaram, G. S.; London, R.; Manimekalai, S., et al. "A-Tocopherol and Serum Lipoproteins." *Lipids*, 1981, *16*, 223-227.

Sunderam, G. S.; London, R.; Margolis, et al. "Serum Hormones and Lipoproteins in Benign Breast Disease." *Cancer Research*, 1981, *41*, 3814-3816.

Tamura, T.; Shane, B.; Baer, M. "Absorption of mono- and polyglutamyl Folates in Zinc-Depleted Man. *American Journal of Clinical Nutrition*, 1978, *31*, 1984-1987.

Terezhalmy, G. T.; Bottomley, W. K.; Pelleu, G. B. "The Use of Water-Soluble Bioflavinoid-Ascorbic Acid Complex in the Treatment of Recurrent Herpes Labialis." *Oral Surgery*, 1978, *45*, 56-62.

Thind, S. K. "Role of B-6 in Oxalate Metabolism in Urolithiasis." *American Journal of Clinical Nutrition*, 1979; (June) 32, xx (abstracts).

Thom, J, A., Morris, J. E.: Bishop, A. "The Influence of Refined Carbohydrate on Urinary Calcium Excretion." *British Journal of Urology*, 1978, *50*, 459-464.

Thornton, J. R. "Diet and Gallstones. *Gut,* 1983, 24, 2-6.

Thorp, V. J. "Effect of Oral Contraceptive Agents on Vitamin and Mineral Requirements." *Journal of the American Dietetic Association*, 1980, *76*, 581-584.

Underwood, E. J. *Trace Elements in Human and Animal Nutrition.* New York: Academic Press, 1977.

U.S. Department of Agriculture, *Nationwide Food Consumption Survey, 1977-78, Preliminary Report No. 2.* Washington, DC, 1980.

U.S. Department of Health, Education and Welfare, "Ten State Nutrition Survey, 1968-70." DHEW Pub. # (HSM) 72-8134, 1971, vols 1-5.

U. S. Department of Health, Education and Welfare, Pub. No. (ADM) 74-124, 1974.

Van Thiel, D. H.; Gavaler, J.; Lester, R. "Ethanol Inhibition of Vitamin A Metabolism in the Testes: Possible Mechanism for Sterility in Alcoholics." *Science*, 1974, *186*, 941-944.

Van Thiel, D. H.; Lester, R. "Sex and Alcohol." *New England Journal of Medicine, 1974, 291*, 251-253.

Wallace, A. M.; Grant, J. K. "Effect of Zinc on Androgen Metabolism in the Human Hyperplastic Prostate." *Biochemical Society Transactions*, 1975, *3*, 540-542.

Walravens, P. A. "Zinc Metabolism and Its Implications in Clinical Medicine." *The Western Journal of Medicine*, 1979, *130*, 133-142.

Wassertheil-Smoller, S.; Romney, S. L.; Wylie-Rosett, J. "Dietary Vitamin C and Uterine Cervical Dysplasia." *American Journal of Epidemology*, 1981, *114*, 714-724.

Weber, F. "Biochemical Mechanisms of Vitamin A Action." *Proceedings of the Nutrition Society*, 1983, 42, 31-41.

White, H. S. "Zinc Content and the Zinc-to-Calorie Ratio of Weighed Diets." *Journal of American Dietetic Association,* 1976, 68, 243-245.

Whorton, D.; Krauss, R. M.; Marshall, S.; Milby, T. H. "Infertility in Male Pesticide Workers." *The Lancet*, 1977, December 17: 1259-1261.

Wolf, G. "Is Dietary Beta-Carotene an Anti-Cancer Agent?" *Nutrition Reviews*, 1982, *40*, 257-261.

Wu, S. H.; Oldfield, J. E.; Whanger, P.D.; Weswig, P. H. "Effect of Selenium, Vitamin E, and Antioxidants on Testicular Function in Rats." *Biology of Reproduction*, 1973, *8*, 625-629.

INDEX